stay fit,
stay young

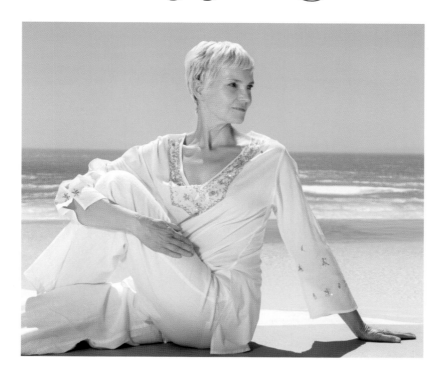

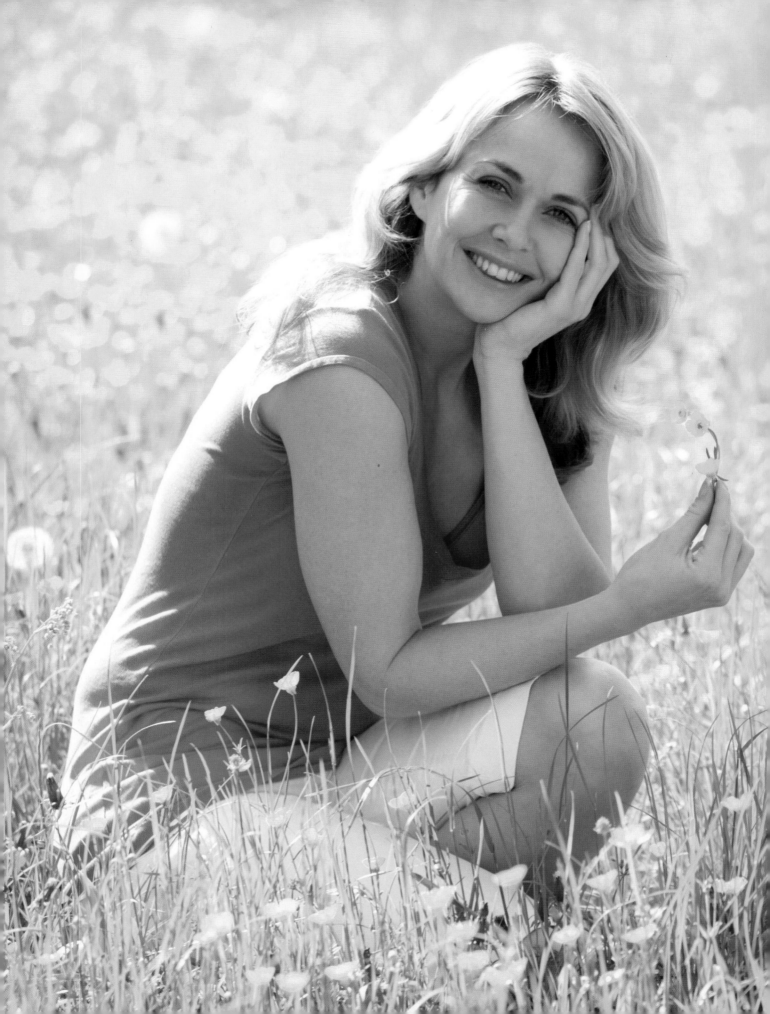

stay fit,
stay young

Easy-to-follow exercises to keep you fit and healthy

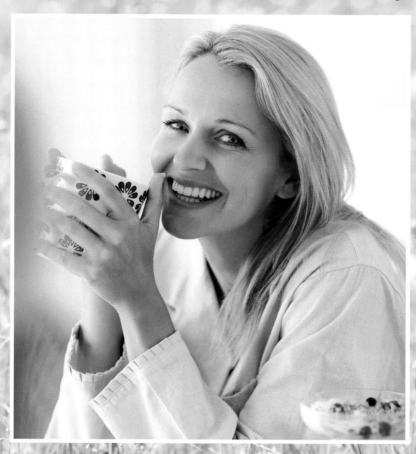

PaRragon

Bath · New York · Singapore · Hong Kong · Cologne · Delhi
Melbourne · Amsterdam · Johannesburg · Auckland · Shenzhen

First published by Parragon in 2010

Parragon
Queen Street House
4 Queen Street
Bath BA1 1HE, UK

Copyright © Parragon Books Ltd 2010

ISBN: 978-1-4454-0641-1

Printed in Indonesia

Produced by Stonecastle Graphics
Designed by Sue Pressley and Paul Turner
Compiled from text by Sara Rose, Faye Rowe, Lucy Wyndham-Read,
    and Kevin Pressley
Edited by Philip de Ste. Croix
Photography by Roddy Paine
Models: Kylie Cushman, Helen Goldthorpe, and Elise Gourbin

Disclaimer

Neither the publisher nor the author is engaged in rendering professional advice or services to the individual reader. The ideas, procedures, and suggestions in this book are not intended as a substitute for consulting with a physician. All matters regarding health require medical supervision. If you have any health problems or medical conditions, consult with your physician before undertaking any of the instructions in this book. Neither the author nor the publisher shall be liable or responsible for any loss or damage allegedly arising from any information or suggestion in this book.

Photo credits

(a = above, b = below, r = right, l = left, c = center)
All photographs © Roddy Paine Photography unless otherwise stated.
© Getty Images: DK Stock/Bruce Talbot 18*al*; Fuse 6*ar*; Jose Luis Pelaez Inc. 19*al*.
© shutterstock.com: Yuri Arcurs 1, 3, 9*b*, 10*a*, 11*bl*, 16*ar*, 17, 19*b*, 23; Monkey Business Images 2–3*l*, 6*bl*, 7*ar*, 7*bl*, 8*a*, 9*a*, 14*ar*, 14*bl*; Objectsforall 16*bc*; Payless Images 8*b*; Piotr Marcinski 19*cr*; Studio37 21*ar*; Zulufoto 10*b*.

Contents

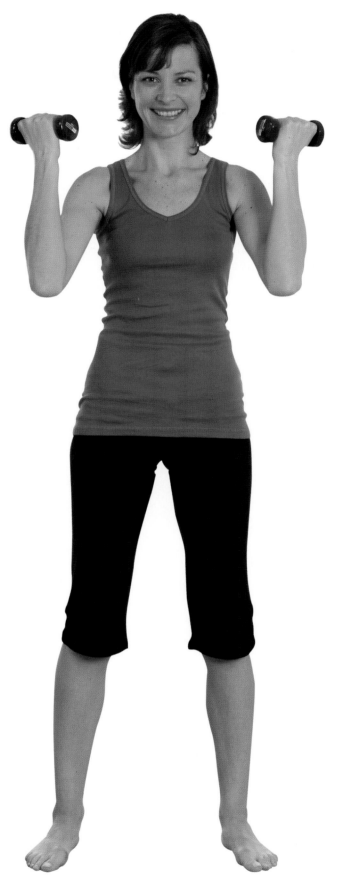

STAYING YOUNG

If you want to keep fit and stay young but dislike the idea of living in the gym or becoming a diet-book bore, don't despair. By following a varied and sensible diet, getting enough sleep and relaxation, and working out using the easy exercises in this book, you'll soon feel healthier and look younger—with more energy and a trimmer figure.

Great reasons for shaping up

Apart from the obvious benefit of improving your appearance, firming and toning up your body is actually good for your health. Strengthening your muscles will improve your balance and posture, and increase your flexibility, helping to keep your body in tip-top condition as you get older. As an added bonus, you'll find it easier to control your weight, because muscles burn more calories than fat.

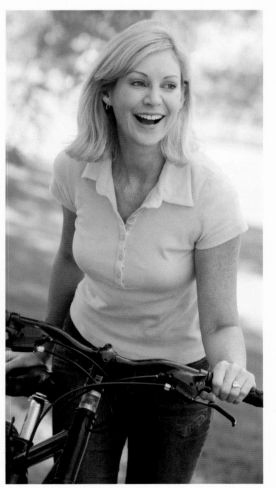

Lifestyle

As you embark on your plan to stay fit and young, it is worth considering making positive changes to your lifestyle to maximize the results of exercising, especially if you're looking for a quick result because you need to look great for a special occasion. Adopting a healthy eating program is the perfect partner to a more active lifestyle; but remember, always speak to your physician or a nutritionist before you make fundamental changes to your diet.

Simply by making healthy food choices—cutting down on fat and sugar, eating lots of fresh fruit and vegetables and drinking at least four pints of water a day—will help to flush toxins out of your system and make your body a more efficient machine so your muscles respond better to exercising. As you begin to exercise regularly, you will slowly start to see your body becoming more toned and fit-looking until you achieve the results you desire.

After two or three weeks you may find that your clothes start to feel a little looser and that your muscles start to look more defined. Some people take a little longer to respond to exercise for a whole range of reasons, such as body composition—whether you naturally have more muscle mass—or other lifestyle factors, but once you've got used to the routine of exercising, it will become second nature and, hopefully, an enjoyable part of your life. Many studies have shown that exercise can be addictive, due to the rush of feel-good chemicals—serotonin and dopamine—that are released in the brain when you work out.

Above: Whatever your age, you will get fitter and feel younger when you adopt a healthier lifestyle and a regular exercise routine.

Left: You will soon find that you have more energy to enjoy life.

Feeling fitter, looking younger

The food we eat and the type of exercise we take have a direct influence on our health and general well-being. The body requires food to build its essential tissues and to create the energy needed to maintain breathing, heart rate, digestion, growth, and repair. Even after we are fully grown and mature, our entire bodies are replaced cell by cell over a period of seven years. The process is complex, but continued damage to replacement cells is thought by scientists to result in aging. Good nutrition will help to give the body the fuel it needs to create healthy new cells and an active lifestyle will maintain the body's strength and ability to function properly.

Health and vitality

Eating sensibly means ensuring your food contains a careful balance of protein, fat, carbohydrates, vitamins, minerals, and water. Together with regular exercise, a sensible eating routine will ensure a healthy mind and body, with higher levels of energy, and a general sense of confidence and vitality. Eat the right food and your body will reward you with clear skin, shiny hair, sparkling

HEALTHY EATING FOR A SLIMMER APPEARANCE

Eating sensibly is essential to maintain good health, but what you actually consume can directly affect the appearance of your stomach, which is often one of the first areas where we notice the addition of a few extra pounds. To look and feel slimmer, keep bloating to a minimum by combining a simple exercise routine with a healthy eating plan. It sounds unlikely, but drinking more water will help you to gain a flatter stomach and reduce bloating as water flushes out toxins and helps to curb your appetite.

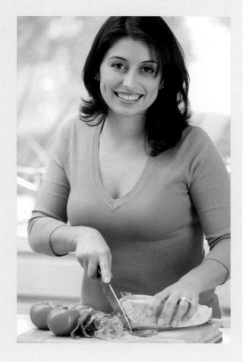

Right: A balanced diet will contain all the vitamins and minerals your body needs.

eyes, and greater resistance to common ailments such as colds and flu. You really are what you eat and a gradual change in your eating habits to include more fresh fruit and vegetables (high in vitamins and minerals) and low-fat sources of protein and carbohydrates will ensure that your body has the right fuel to create energy. To maintain a healthy diet you need to eat foods from the five main food groups: bread, cereals, and potatoes (carbohydrates); fruit and vegetables; milk and dairy products; meat, fish, and alternatives (proteins) and foods containing fat or sugar.

There is no need to change your eating habits overnight. Changes are best made gradually until healthy eating habits replace old bad habits. Swap that afternoon chocolate bar for a nice juicy apple and replace that fizzy drink with water or fruit juice and your body will soon notice the benefits. Simple changes, such as choosing whole wheat bread instead of white processed loaves, are easy to make without upsetting your usual routine.

Left: Sensible food choices will benefit the whole family.

A balanced diet

As well as vitamins, minerals, and trace elements, the body requires certain other elements in order to make repairs and create energy.

Protein: About one fifth of the adult body is made up of proteins which are essential building blocks for body maintenance and cell repair. Protein is present in different forms and quantities in many foods. Some protein-rich foods such as red meat, eggs, cheese, and nuts are also high in fat while others such as fish, beans, and peas are low in fat.

Fats: Important for a wide range of body functions, fats and oils provide a valuable source of energy in the form of calories. Fats are classified as either saturated, monounsaturated, or polyunsaturated. Saturated fats are usually solid at room temperature (e.g. butter) and are believed to raise the level of harmful LDL (low-density lipoprotein) cholesterol connected to heart disease. Polyunsaturated fats reduce both HDL (high-density lipoprotein) and LDL cholesterol. The omega-3 fatty acids (found in oily fish) are believed to reduce the risk of heart disease. Monounsaturated fats raise the ratio of beneficial HDL to LDL and may also have a protective role in the prevention of coronary heart disease.

Carbohydrate: Essential for instant energy, carbohydrate is vital fuel for muscle contraction, although excess carbohydrates not immediately needed for energy are stored in the body as fat. Valuable sources include pasta, bread, potatoes, rice, and other grains.

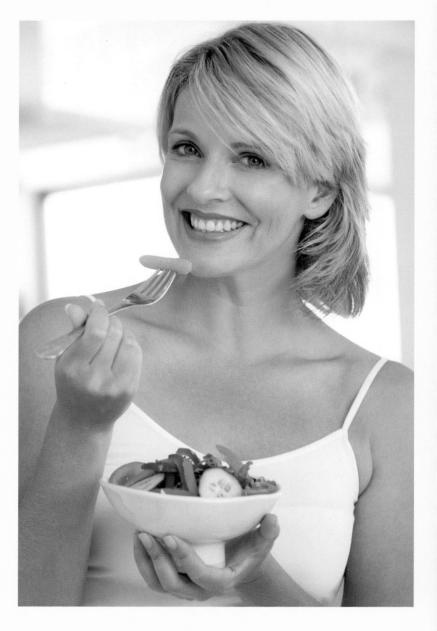

Above: A balanced diet will provide all the nutrition your body needs for energy and a healthier, more youthful appearance.

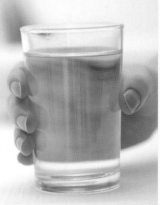

WATER

Drink at least eight glasses (four pints) of water a day (but don't drink large amounts before exercising or you'll put pressure on your bladder). To make sure you're drinking enough water, check the color of your urine—the paler it is, the better. If your body feels deprived of water then it will hold on to what there is, which can lead to water retention and the appearance of bloating.

Fiber: The fibrous parts of natural plant foods are not absorbed by the body and remain in the intestine after digestion. Fiber is vital for the bowel to function normally and is known to help lower blood fats (lipids), helping to reduce the risk of heart disease. Fiber provides a satisfying bulk to meals without added fat or calories. Fruit and vegetables—complete with their skins—are very high in fiber. Other good sources are whole grain cereals, whole wheat bread and pasta, brown rice, beans, and lentils. Processed foods such as white bread and white pasta have had the fiber removed.

Essential vitamins and minerals

These are the main vitamins and minerals you need to include in a balanced diet.

Vitamin A (Retinol): Necessary for normal vision and to maintain healthy skin and surface tissues. Found in meat—particularly liver, fish oils, dairy produce, egg yolk, beets, and artichoke.

Vitamin B complex (B1, B2, B3, B5, B6, B12): All B vitamins are essential for correct functioning of the brain, digestive, and nervous systems and for healthy skin, hair, eyes, mouth, and liver. Protects against mild depression and anemia. To be found in yeast, liver, pork, cereals, beans, peas, nuts, kidney, lamb, beef, leeks, spinach, parsnips, celery, broccoli, milk, fruit, potatoes, and bananas.

Vitamin C (Ascorbic acid): Assists in growth and repair of cells and tissues. Fights infection and is essential for effective absorption of iron. To be found in vegetables and fruit, especially citrus fruits, blackcurrants, guavas, broccoli, and rose hips.

Vitamin D (Cholecalciferol): Needed for the absorption of calcium into the blood and maintenance of healthy bones and teeth. To be found in eggs, butter, cheese, milk, oily fish, liver, and generated by natural sunlight.

Folate (Folic acid): Essential for cell growth, especially in pregnancy. To be found in offal, yeast extract, and green leafy vegetables.

Calcium: Essential for the maintenance of bones and connective tissue. Deficiency may accelerate osteoporosis. Best sources are milk, cheese, and yogurt. Also occurs in fruits, vegetables, and seeds.

Iron: Essential for the prevention of anemia. Present in a wide range of foods, especially proteins—red meat such as liver, dairy foods, and egg yolk. Also found in oysters, raisins, chocolate, molasses, and dried apricots.

Zinc: Helps wound healing and enzyme activity. Present in a wide range of foods, especially proteins—meat and dairy foods.

EAT WELL

Look and feel better with these healthy eating tips:

• Choose a wide selection of fresh fruit and vegetables.

• Eat little and often and make sure you consume a varied diet. Keep wheat products to a minimum as they cause bloating, giving the appearance of a large stomach and making you feel uncomfortable.

• Sit down to eat and chew thoroughly. It takes 15 minutes for your brain to receive a message from your stomach telling you that it's full, so if you eat too quickly you are liable to overeat because that crucial "full" message will not have reached the brain in time.

• Reduce the amount of saturated fat you consume.

• Don't eat too many starchy carbohydrates, such as rice, bread, potatoes and pasta. They're low in fiber (which means you will want to eat more, more often) and are stored mostly as fat.

• Say goodbye to fizzy drinks—even if they're labeled as caffeine-free or "diet," they still cause bloating because they're loaded with additives.

• Avoid processed food and ready meals—they are laden with salt, sugar, and chemicals and they upset your stomach's bacterial balance.

• Reduce salt—it causes fluid retention and can have health implications.

• Limit your intake of cookies, candy, and cakes—they give an instant sugar rush rather than sustained energy levels, and promote cravings for more food.

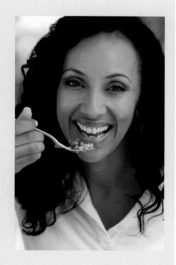

Above: Fresh unprocessed foods are packed full of vitamins.

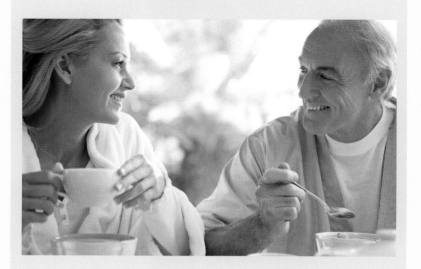

Above: *A healthy eating plan will give you more energy to enjoy life.*

BODY BASICS

The exercises in this book have been chosen to help you tone up all over, so you'll get balanced results. They are divided into different sections: standing, seated, and floor exercises and each exercise identifies which main area of the body is being worked. If you have a quick look through the book, you will find exercises devoted to targeting shoulders, arms, chest, stomach, thighs, and buttocks. Each exercise is carefully explained with step-by-step instructions.

Many of the exercises also work your core muscles, such as those found deep within the torso. This helps to develop your core stability, which will help to prevent injury during exercise and correct your posture. Exercises that work your core stability, such as the abdominal curl on page 72, require you to "engage" your stomach muscles. You can do this by pulling in your stomach muscles toward your spine, being careful not to hold your breath. This should automatically cause you to stand or lie in a straight line and create the perfect starting position to carry out the exercise.

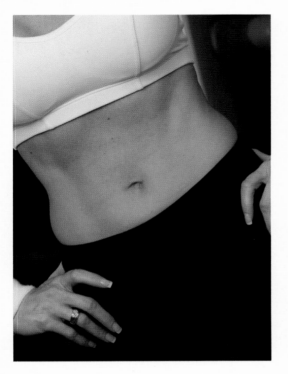

The exercises

Before starting the exercise plan you should seek advice from your physician, especially if you are pregnant or suffer from back pain, in order to rule out any reason why it wouldn't be suitable for you. Most of the exercises in this book are easy to do, but if you do find any exercises particularly difficult to carry out, then you should stop attempting to do them and seek advice from a qualified fitness expert before carrying on. The most important thing to remember is that it's better to work in your comfort zone, rather than push yourself too hard. It's also important to remember that even when an exercise requires you to fully extend your arms or legs, you keep your knees and elbows "soft" (slightly bent) to help guard against possible injury.

It is very helpful to have a basic understanding of how your body works, and why it's important to have good posture, before you embark on an exercise routine. Being muscle-aware will help you to target the areas that you want to firm up.

Above: If you are new to exercising, do not attempt to do too many exercises at one time. As your fitness improves, you will be able to work out for longer.

Left: The core muscles give your body stability and enable you to perform a wide range of everyday movements.

How your body moves

Your body's framework is the skeleton, made up of more than 200 bones that support your muscles and allow you to move. Muscles fixed to the ends of bones permit an enormous range of movement. However, joints and muscles that are not regularly exercised may become stiff and immobile, leading to pain and possible injury.

Muscles are made up of millions of tiny protein filaments that relax and contract to produce movement. Most muscles are attached to bones by tendons and are consciously controlled by your brain. Movement happens when muscles pull on tendons, which move the bones at the joints. Most movements require the coordinated use of several muscle groups.

Posture

The alignment of your muscles and joints is known as posture. If your posture is consistently poor over a period of time, your muscles will be subjected to uneven stresses, leading to aching muscles and joints, tiredness, weakness, and an increased risk of injury when exercising.

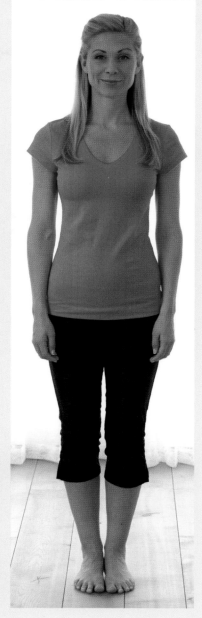

Good posture looks natural and relaxed, not slouched and hunched. When you are standing up, your neck should be in line with your spine, with your head balanced squarely on top, your shoulder blades set back and down, and your spine long and curving naturally. Your hips should be straight. Good posture when sitting means sitting up straight with your feet flat on the floor and your lower back supported.

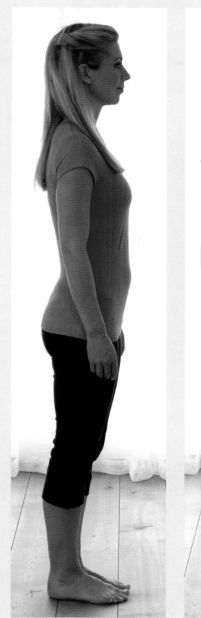

HOW TO CHECK YOUR POSTURE

Stand sideways in front of a full-length mirror to assess your posture. Imagine there is a straight line drawn down the center of your body. If your posture is spot-on, the line will pass through the center of the ear lobe, the tip of the shoulder, halfway through the chest, slightly behind the hip, and just outside the ankle bone.

It does take time to correct any postural deficiencies you may have but it is important to identify what your weaknesses are—for example, rounded shoulders—so that you can work on correcting these. The good news is that by training your core muscles you will be strengthening the muscles that hold up your back and automatically improving your posture.

The spine

The spine is an S-shaped, flexible curve that supports your skull, acts as a structural base to which your limbs, ribs, and pelvis attach, and enables you to stand upright. It also provides movement for your trunk, allowing you to bend forward, backward, and to the side, and twist. The spine has three natural curves: in at the back of the neck, outward at the back of the ribcage, and in again in the lower back (lumbar spine).

To protect your spine, you should aim to maintain its natural curve, particularly in the lumbar region. This is called putting your spine into neutral, and nearly every exercise in this book will require you to do this. It's essential that you can perform this maneuver correctly, so use the instructions on the following pages as a guide to this correct position.

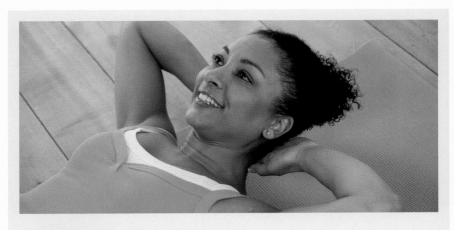

PROTECT YOUR SPINE WHILE EXERCISING

- Be conscious of your neck—it's fine to cradle the sides of your head with your hands, but avoid resting your head on your hands because you may pull on your neck.
- Keep your abdominal muscles pulled in—this will protect your lower spine.
- Exercise on a mat or other padded surface to prevent bruising.
- Always keep your knees slightly bent when performing leg exercises—straight-leg exercising makes your hip flexors pull directly on the spine, causing excessive strain on your lower back.

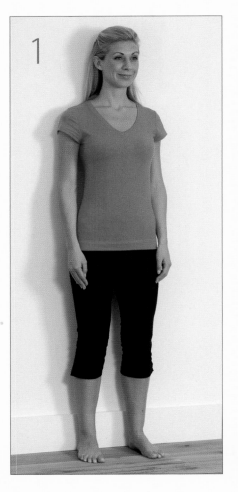

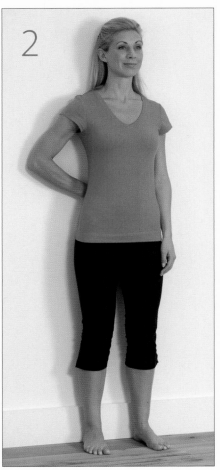

Standing neutral

1 Stand tall against a wall with your buttocks and shoulders touching the wall. Keep your feet parallel and hip-width apart, with your weight evenly distributed over both feet. Gently pull up through your legs, keeping your knees slightly bent, and pull your tailbone down toward the floor.

2 Place your hand between the wall and your lower back. The neutral position is slightly different for everyone, but it should feel comfortable and you should just be able to place the flat of your hand between your back and the wall. If you can only get your fingers through, your back is too flat and your pelvis is tilted too far forward. If you can get your whole hand through, then your back is too arched and your pelvis too far back.

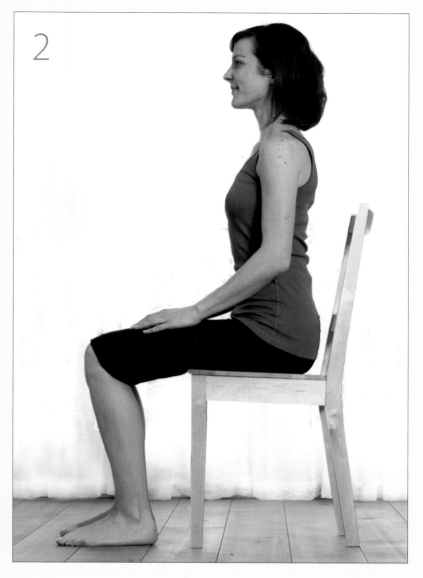

2

Sitting neutral

1 Sit up straight on a stool, chair, or exercise ball with your weight evenly distributed over both buttocks. Keep your feet flat on the floor, and a distance of hip-width apart.

2 Look straight ahead and keep your spine and neck long. Pull your shoulder blades down toward the waist to stop your shoulders from hunching or slumping forward.

3 The natural curves at your neck and your waist should be evident.

Lying down neutral

1 Lie down on your back with your knees bent and your feet flat on the floor, hip-width apart. Your spine will be flat against the floor, apart from the curve of the neck and the lower back.

2 Press your waist back onto the floor by tilting your pelvis back so that you lose the curve in your lower back. Now tilt your pelvis forward so that your lower back over-arches. Then find the midpoint between these two extremes. You should be able to slip one hand under your waist and feel a slight gap between your back and the floor.

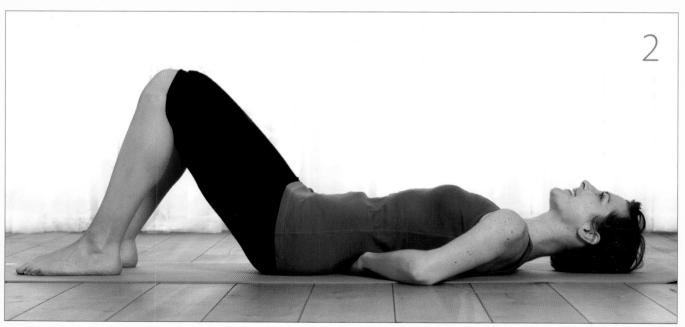

2

Core muscles

The core of your body is simply what's between the shoulders and hips—basically, the trunk and pelvis. The core is a crucial group of muscles, not only for sports, but also for normal daily activities as well, because it comes into play just about every time you move.

The core acts to produce force (for example, during lifting), it stabilizes the body to permit other musculature to produce force (for example, during running), and it's also called upon to transfer energy (for example, during jumping). This is why it is so important that your core is fit and strong. Your balance and coordination will be improved, and, most important of all, the stability that these muscles bring will help to keep your spine healthy and flexible.

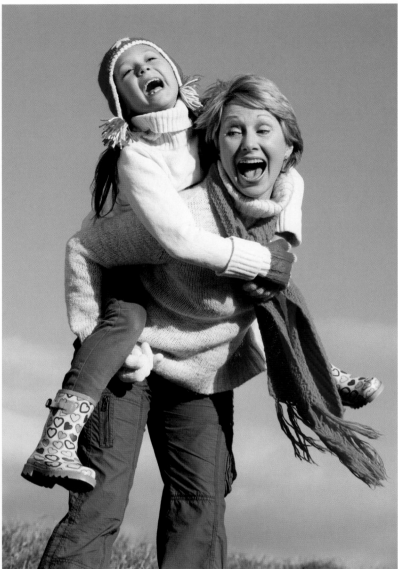

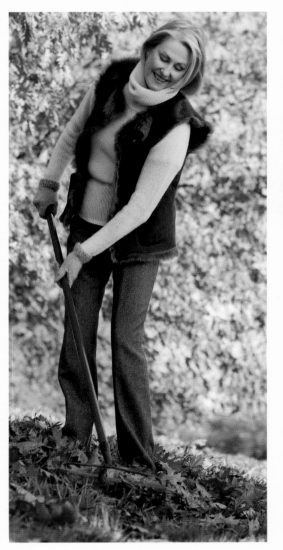

What is core stability?

Core stability is the effective use of the core muscles to help stabilize the spine, allowing your limbs to move more freely. Good core stability means you can keep your mid-section rigid without forces such as gravity affecting your movements. The positive effects of this include reducing the chance of injury, better posture, increased agility and flexibility, and improved coordination.

Core stability is necessary for everyday life, not just for sport. To pick up a child, for example, requires a core strength in order not only to lift the child but also to do it in a safe and efficient way that avoids you injuring yourself.

Above: Good core stability creates strength and improves flexibility.

Left: The core muscles enable you to perform a wide range of everyday movements.

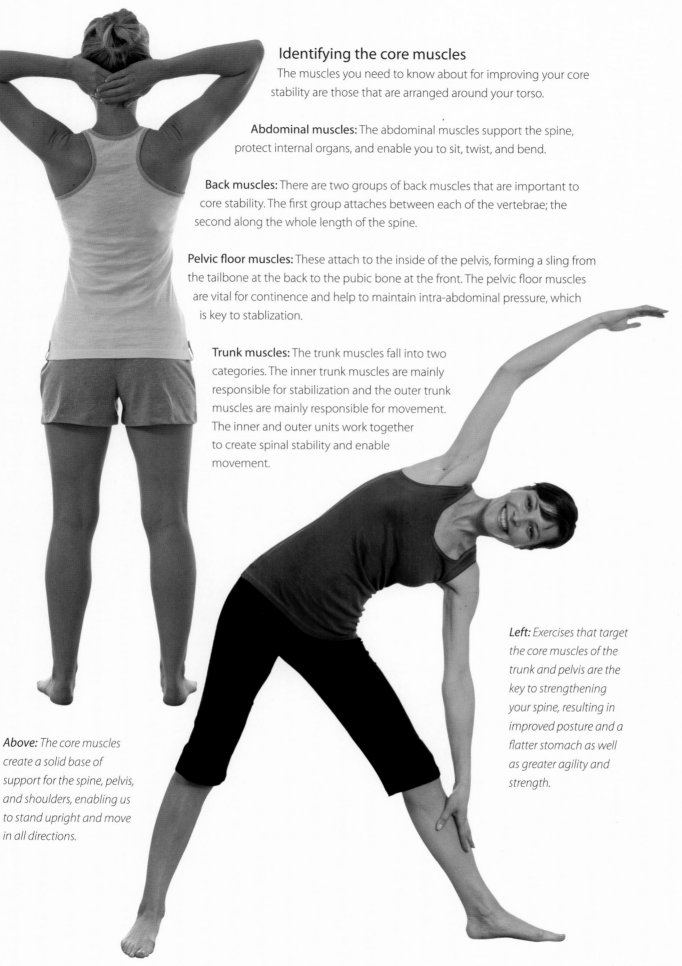

Identifying the core muscles

The muscles you need to know about for improving your core stability are those that are arranged around your torso.

Abdominal muscles: The abdominal muscles support the spine, protect internal organs, and enable you to sit, twist, and bend.

Back muscles: There are two groups of back muscles that are important to core stability. The first group attaches between each of the vertebrae; the second along the whole length of the spine.

Pelvic floor muscles: These attach to the inside of the pelvis, forming a sling from the tailbone at the back to the pubic bone at the front. The pelvic floor muscles are vital for continence and help to maintain intra-abdominal pressure, which is key to stablization.

Trunk muscles: The trunk muscles fall into two categories. The inner trunk muscles are mainly responsible for stabilization and the outer trunk muscles are mainly responsible for movement. The inner and outer units work together to create spinal stability and enable movement.

Above: The core muscles create a solid base of support for the spine, pelvis, and shoulders, enabling us to stand upright and move in all directions.

Left: Exercises that target the core muscles of the trunk and pelvis are the key to strengthening your spine, resulting in improved posture and a flatter stomach as well as greater agility and strength.

GETTING STARTED

A good way to start is to spend a quiet afternoon looking through this book to help familiarize yourself with the various stretches and exercises. Each exercise is explained with step-by-step instructions, and is clearly illustrated. Once you've changed into your comfortable clothes, you should switch off the television or any telephones and put on some soothing music to help get you in the mood.

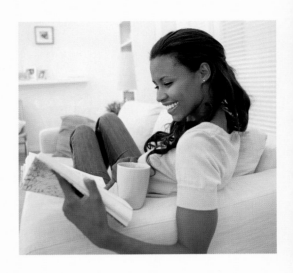

Your workout space

Designate an uncluttered space in your home that is warm and well ventilated and large enough for you to extend your arms and legs without knocking anything over. Ideally, there will be enough space to enable you to take at least five steps in all directions. An exercise mat is a good idea to cushion your body when doing floor work. If possible, try to do your exercise routine in front of a full-length mirror so that you can keep an eye on what you are doing.

What you need

Wear several layers of comfortable clothing as you start to exercise to warm up your muscles, and gradually strip off some of these layers as you get warmer. Clothes should be loose, soft, and made from a breathable fabric—shorts and a vest covered with jogging bottoms and a sweatshirt, for example, are ideal.

There is no need to invest in expensive gym equipment, but it is a good idea to use a nonslip padded exercise mat for safety and to prevent discomfort and bruising. Some of the exercises can be performed using a set of small dumbbells or hand weights to increase the level of difficulty, but do not use weights if you are new to exercising or have back problems. A few of the exercises in this book use an exercise ball and you can find out more about exercise balls on page 22.

How to use this book

The key to a toned body, increased fitness, and more energy is to exercise little but often. Aim to exercise three or four times a week. You'll feel the benefits even if you can only manage ten minutes at a time. As you become fitter and stronger, you'll find that you can easily increase the intensity and the length of time of your workout.

To start with, aim to do each exercise five times, but remember that it is the quality of the movement that is important, not the quantity. Start gently and build up the number of exercises as you become fitter, until you can perform ten repetitions. Don't attempt to do too much too soon. This book has a variety of easy exercises that are designed to work all areas of the body, enabling you to create workout plans to target specific areas of the body and slot a workout into even your busiest day. Exercises are grouped into suggested workouts at the end of the book, but you can mix and match to create your own for even more variety.

Above: Look through the exercises before you begin your first workout.

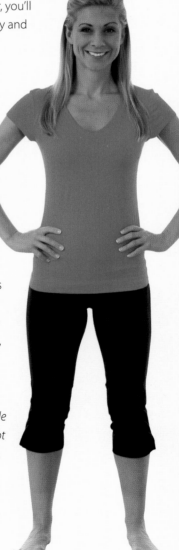

Right: Wear comfortable loose clothes that do not restrict your movement.

Left and above left: Small dumbbells and a nonslip exercise mat are good investments.

WARM UP AND STRETCH

Warming up is very important—if you don't warm up you are likely to injure yourself because your muscles, tendons, and ligaments will be taut. Always make sure you are warm before you stretch, so take a brisk walk around your home or march on the spot for a few seconds to help get your muscles into gear. You should always do this general warm-up, especially if you've just jumped out of bed in the morning. Begin your routine with some gentle stretching and avoid the danger of pulling any muscles by sticking to what you're comfortable doing.

One golden rule to consider while stretching is that you should try to do each one to the best of your ability, but you should never push yourself so far that you feel any pain. We suggest you hold all the stretches in this book for a maximum of three sets of ten seconds, but always take care not to overdue things, particularly if you are new to exercising. It can be tempting to "bounce" while in the stretch to try to get down even farther if you are reaching for the floor, for example. However, this can strain the muscles, and should be avoided. If, once you've got used to stretching, you feel that you could improve your performance, you can try to increase the stretch by slowly and gently moving farther into position. If you ever develop a persistent pain as a result of doing the stretches, make sure you see your medical practitioner for advice.

It is just as important to cool down after your exercise session as it is to warm up before you begin. As well as helping to prevent dizziness and a sudden drop in body temperature, cooling down and stretching gently realigns working muscles to their normal position in order to avoid potential tightness and stiffness.

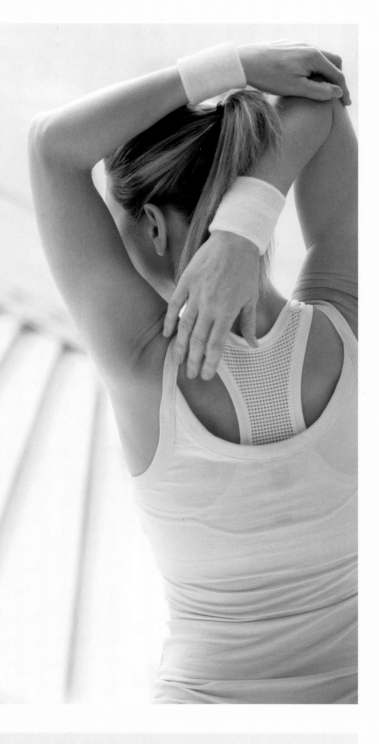

GOOD PRACTICE

Before you begin:

- Drink at least four pints of water a day to make sure you are well hydrated (but don't drink too much before exercising).
- Make sure your practice area is clear and you are unlikely to be interrupted.
- Relax. Don't start the session if you are feeling tense.
- Warm up properly.

After your session:

- Make sure you cool down properly.
- Have a shower or go for a leisurely walk after you have finished your session to help you make the transition back to your normal activity—do not just stop moving.
- Do not go straight to bed if you are exercising at the end of the day.

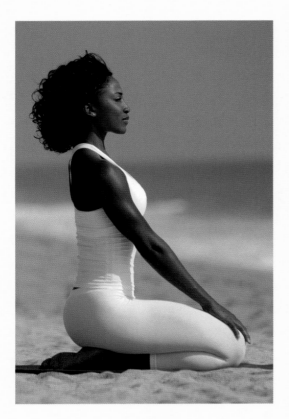

Breathing

It sounds silly, but you must remember to breathe at all times. Correct breathing comes from the deepest area of the lungs, and benefits both your body and mind. But years of stress and poor lifestyle have left most of us with shallow, rapid breathing, whereby we use only the top third of our lungs.

Many people have a tendency to hold their breath as they hold certain poses, which isn't advisable. Make sure that you breathe deeply and slowly throughout the routine, because it will help to deliver oxygen to the muscles and make the exercises more effective. The correct way to breathe when exercising is to breathe in slowly through your nose (notice how your abdominal cavity rises as you do so), and breathe out slowly through your mouth. Make sure you continue to breathe in and out regularly throughout an exercise. And don't hold your breath—this will cause your blood pressure to rise, which can be dangerous.

Left: If you are breathing correctly, the chest and diaphram should expand as you inhale, filling the lungs, and contract as you exhale, pushing the air out of the body.

Below: If you are new to exercising, begin with five repetitions of each exercise. As your body becomes used to exercise and your muscles grow stronger, you will be able to perform a greater number of repetitions with ease.

Controlling your movements

All exercises should be done slowly and in a meditative fashion. Concentrate on what you're doing, and think about how your body is responding to each exercise. If any action feels quick or jerky, or hurts, you're not doing it properly. Each movement should flow in a slow, gentle manner. This lets your muscles warm up and stretch naturally. It takes time to learn a more gentle approach to movement, but if you try to keep your body relaxed as you move, with practice your body will become used to performing the exercises naturally.

Reps and sets

Muscle-building exercises are done as a series of repetitions (reps). One repetition equals one exercise. A set is usually a group of ten repetitions but may consist of anything between five and 15 reps, depending on your level of fitness. The aim of repeating exercises is to work until your muscles feel tired, and over time this will strengthen them so that they can work even harder. It's important that you don't stop for more than a minute between exercises. Shorter recovery periods result in better muscles all round and improved muscle endurance. So keep going!

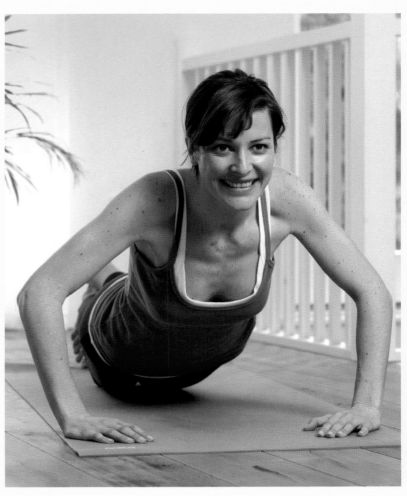

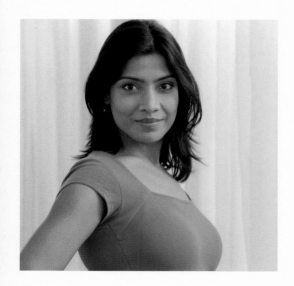

The effects of toning

After a few weeks of exercise and a healthy eating routine, one of the biggest changes you will notice in yourself is in performance. It depends how fit you already are when you start this program, but you should gradually be able to increase the number of reps of each exercise you can manage. Some women worry that if they do toning exercises for their upper body they will bulk up. This is simply not true—women do not have enough testosterone to build large muscles. You would have to be lifting heavy weights and following a strict strength-training workout for your muscles to bulk up!

MORNING EXERCISE

If you are not previously used to exercising, doing just a few minutes exercise three or four times a week will add up to a fair bit and you could notice quite dramatic effects, such as weight loss and having firmer, more toned muscles. If you have enough time, doing these exercises in the morning is a great way to kick start your day as this will speed up your metabolic rate and you will burn off more calories. You will also feel virtuous for the rest of the day knowing you have done your exercises! But, if you find that you're struggling to make time for exercise in the morning, try these top tips:

• Visualize how your body will look and how you will feel if you stick religiously to your plan. It will help you to realize why doing the exercises regularly is essential.

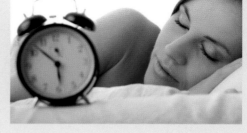

• Try setting your alarm half an hour earlier than you usually do so that you can exercise in the morning—you can have an extra ten-minute lie-in and still have time to enjoy some exercise.

• Invest in some flattering sportswear—it will make you want to jump out of bed just to wear it.

Above: Make time for exercise in the morning.

• Start the day with a cup of warm water and a slice of lemon—it will help to detox your system and focus your mind.

• Try playing some upbeat, motivating music while you do the routine.

Above: You will soon notice how much more energy you have and how toned your body has become.

Right: Whatever your age, you will soon feel the benefits of regular exercise and a healthier diet, including increased vitality, glowing skin, and a slimmer, healthier appearance.

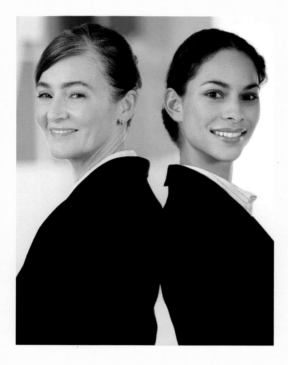

The long-term benefits of exercise

Over time, your fitness, strength, and stamina will all improve and your movements will become more fluid and graceful. Exercise is excellent for reducing stress—controlled movement and stretching encourages greater relaxation, particularly when combined with mental focus and a good breathing technique.

Nearly everyone can benefit from an exercise routine tailored to their own level of fitness. Even if you haven't exercised for years or have recently had a baby, you can start by doing a few stretches and gradually make your workout more challenging as your strength and level of overall fitness improve. Go to page 92 where you will find some workout suggestions using the exercises in this book.

Mental focus

To feel the full benefit of each exercise, you need to approach each one with good mental focus. A strong connection between mind and body will bring about positive effects on your body, both internally and externally. By concentrating on how and where you are moving, you are more likely to move correctly and safely.

Relax the mind and body

When your body and mind are under stress your muscles become constricted, restricting the blood supply and dramatically affecting the way that your body functions. One of the simplest ways to relax is to use a technique called "progressive muscle relaxation," which tenses and releases all the major muscle groups. Lie down, close your eyes, and concentrate on breathing slowly. Tense and release the muscles in each foot, then loosen and relax it. Work your way systematically up your body from your toes to your head, tensing and releasing each muscle group. Try this before you start your exercise workout.

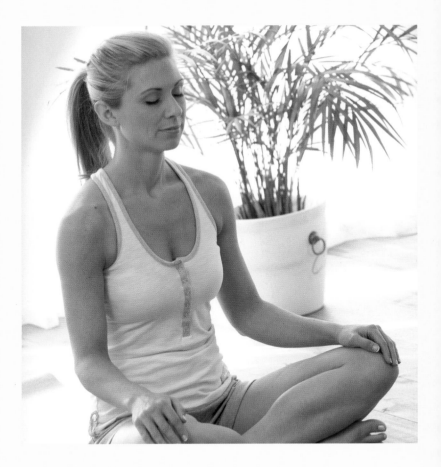

RELAXATION TECHNIQUE

Lie down on your back with your legs either bent or straight (whatever is most comfortable) and place a small cushion or folded towel underneath your head. Place your hands at your sides. Begin to focus on your breathing. Breathe deeply into the body, through the chest, ribcage, and down to into the abdomen. Inhale through the nose and exhale through the mouth.
As you breathe, allow your body to relax and any tension to release into the floor.
Deepen the breathing.

- Inhale for 4 counts, exhale for 4 counts. Repeat 6 times.
- Inhale for 4 counts, exhale for 6 counts. Repeat 6 times.
- Inhale for 4 counts, exhale for 8 counts. Repeat 6 times.
- Inhale for 4 counts, hold for 2 counts, exhale for 8 counts, hold for 2 counts.

Continue to breathe at this pace for 5–10 minutes. If your mind wanders, bring the focus back to the breath. People have different responses to relaxation. If this technique does not feel right for you, try visualizing a beautiful place, somewhere you feel safe and relaxed. Imagine yourself there and breathe slowly and rhythmically (see opposite).

Basic visualization

Creating mental pictures that correspond to what you are trying to do in your workout can be enormously useful in helping you to perform the exercise correctly. As you perform each exercise, think about how each part of your body feels and try to visualize these parts. It may take a bit of time to learn the techniques but it's worth the effort.

Perform this simple visualization exercise to relax and calm your mind before you start your workout. Choose a quiet, comfortable place where you won't be disturbed. Sit or lie down and breathe slowly, trying to relax your body. Focus on your chosen mental image—for example, visualize somewhere beautiful outdoors, such as a mountain, park, garden, or an exotic empty beach with clear blue sea and sky—and picture yourself here. At the same time you can repeat positive affirmations such as "I am happy and relaxed." Maintain this image for about ten minutes, breathing slowly and rhythmically as you do so.

Above right: It is worth practicing simple visualization techniques to help you focus and relax.

Opposite above: Relaxation creates a strong connection between mind and body, allowing you to concentrate fully on the effects of the movements on your muscles.

Right: Positive thinking will help you to get the most from your workout.

The power of positive thinking

Using your mind and emotions will help you to get the most from your workout. Use positive thoughts while you are exercising and focus on what you are doing right, rather than what you are getting wrong. Telling yourself that you are doing well can make you do even better, while sending negative messages to yourself sets you up to fail. To get yourself into the right frame of mind, use visualizations and affirmations (making positive statements) such as "My stomach muscles are becoming more toned."

SAY GOODBYE TO STRESS

Stress is something that is increasingly apparent in our daily lives. One of the best ways to beat the effects of stress is to build regular times in your life when you actively choose to do something to relieve it. A regular exercise routine will help to combat stress and restore emotional and physical balance.

USING AN EXERCISE BALL

Exercises that use a ball work on your body's muscle groups from a strong central core. They encourage the use of good breathing techniques, strong mental focus, and smooth, flowing movements. The whole point of using an exercise ball is that it is an unstable base, which makes you work extra muscles—the simple act of sitting on the ball improves postural strength and awareness. Through regular exercise using the ball, your abdominal and spinal muscles, which act as a splint around your spine, will become stronger.

Exercise balls are widely available from sports stores and are not expensive. There are many on the market, varying in color, size, cost, and quality. Be sure to choose one that is strong and burst-resistant, for safety, and is designed to take at least 660 lb (300 kg) in weight: remember that the ball will have to take the combined weight of your body and any weights you may be using during your workouts.

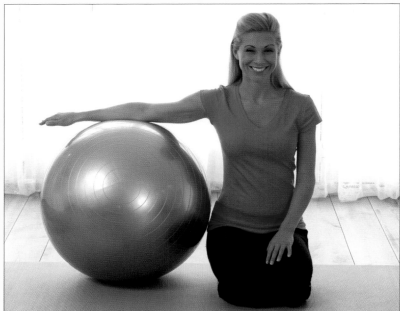

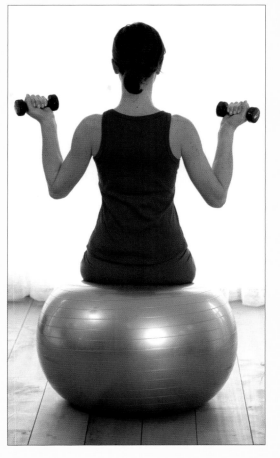

Choosing the right size of ball

It is essential to use the correct size of ball. When you are sitting on your ball, your knees and hips should be at an angle of 90 degrees or greater. Using a ball that is too small or too large makes exercising awkward. The length of your arm from the shoulder to the fingertip is generally a good way to work out which is the right ball for you, but try one out in the store to make sure.

Arm length	Ball size required
22–26 in (55–65 cm)	22 in (55 cm)
26–31.5 in (66–80 cm)	26 in (65 cm)
32–35.5 in (81–90 cm)	30 in (75 cm)
more than 36 in (90 cm)	34 in (85 cm)

Above: Using the correct size of exercise ball will make the exercises more comfortable and effective for you.

Left: Working out with an exercise ball can be fun and is an excellent way to improve how your body looks, feels, and performs.

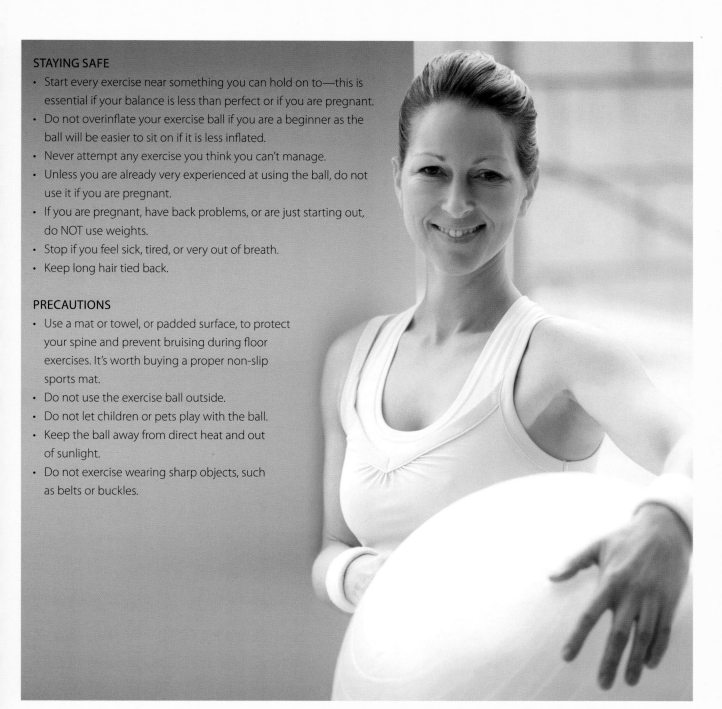

STAYING SAFE

- Start every exercise near something you can hold on to—this is essential if your balance is less than perfect or if you are pregnant.
- Do not overinflate your exercise ball if you are a beginner as the ball will be easier to sit on if it is less inflated.
- Never attempt any exercise you think you can't manage.
- Unless you are already very experienced at using the ball, do not use it if you are pregnant.
- If you are pregnant, have back problems, or are just starting out, do NOT use weights.
- Stop if you feel sick, tired, or very out of breath.
- Keep long hair tied back.

PRECAUTIONS

- Use a mat or towel, or padded surface, to protect your spine and prevent bruising during floor exercises. It's worth buying a proper non-slip sports mat.
- Do not use the exercise ball outside.
- Do not let children or pets play with the ball.
- Keep the ball away from direct heat and out of sunlight.
- Do not exercise wearing sharp objects, such as belts or buckles.

Getting started

Inflate your ball according to the manufacturer's advice using a hand-operated pump so that it is firm, but not tight like a drum, with a little give. A slightly firmer ball makes it harder to stabilize and balance. Choose a safe, nonslip area on which to exercise. Your surroundings should be free of furniture and clutter. Check the floor for objects which could hurt you or damage the exercise ball. If possible, try to exercise in front of a full-length mirror so that you can check what you are doing.

Stay in control

When you're using an exercise ball you need to be in control at all times. Along with focusing your mind, you need to learn how to use your breathing and how to make your movements coordinated, smooth, and flowing. Otherwise, you may strain or injure yourself. Learning to move in a controlled way helps your body reach its potential. With a little practice you will find you can train your mind to exert a greater influence over your body and you'll be doing this automatically.

WARM UP AND STRETCH

You should always warm up to stretch your muscles, tendons, and ligaments before and after exercising, even if you are only doing a short session, otherwise you are likely to injure yourself. Warming up should involve a few minutes of aerobic exercise, such as marching or jogging on the spot, followed by a series of stretches. Hold each stretch for a count of ten if you can. Remember to keep your back straight throughout your warm-up. You should also stretch at the end of your exercises when you cool down to loosen any muscles that may become cramped or tight.

Marching

This general warming-up exercise will help to raise your body temperature and increase blood flow to the muscles before you begin your exercises. March on the spot for at least a minute, swinging your arms and gradually raising your knees higher as you go (but not so that you're goose-stepping). Make sure your breathing is deep and regular as you march. Once you feel warm, take the time to perform a few stretching exercises.

Forward bend

With this exercise, bend only as far as is comfortable—you don't have to touch your toes. Remember, you'll be able to stretch farther as time goes by and you become more supple with regular exercise.

1 Stand up straight with your feet hip-width apart and your knees slightly bent rather than locked and rigid. Place your hands palm downward on the front of your thighs.

2 Tighten your abdominal muscles by gently pulling in your navel toward your backbone.

3 Slowly slide your hands down your legs toward your toes. Try not to over-arch your back.

4 Position yourself so you feel a stretch in the hamstrings at the back of your thighs, but don't stretch so far that it hurts.

5 Hold for a count of three then return to the center. Repeat four more times. Keep your breathing steady throughout.

TOP TIPS FOR SUPER STRETCHING
- Only stretch warm muscles.
- Slowly ease the muscle into position.
- Do not bounce into position.
- Never overstretch—mild discomfort is acceptable but, if it hurts, you should stop.
- Don't hold your breath.

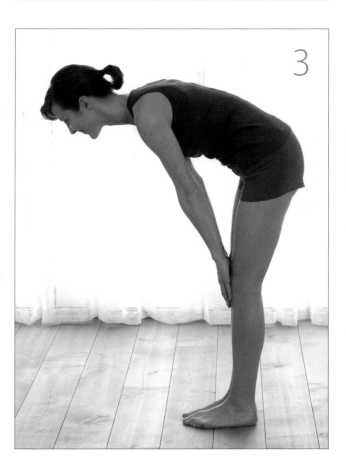

back

Cat stretch

This stretch is known as the Cat stretch because you look a lot like a cat if you do it right! It targets most of the major muscles in the back.

1 Get down on the floor on all fours. Let your head and neck relax so they are in line with your spine and you are looking down toward the floor.

2 Slowly arch your back, by pulling in your stomach muscles and pushing the curve of your spine toward the ceiling. Tilt your head and neck up toward the ceiling as you do this.

3 Hold the stretch for around eight seconds then lower your back so it's straight and in the starting position again. While you do this, let your head and neck relax also. Pause for a brief moment then repeat three times.

4 When you have finished, lean back on to your heels and stretch your arms out in front of you—this completes the movement.

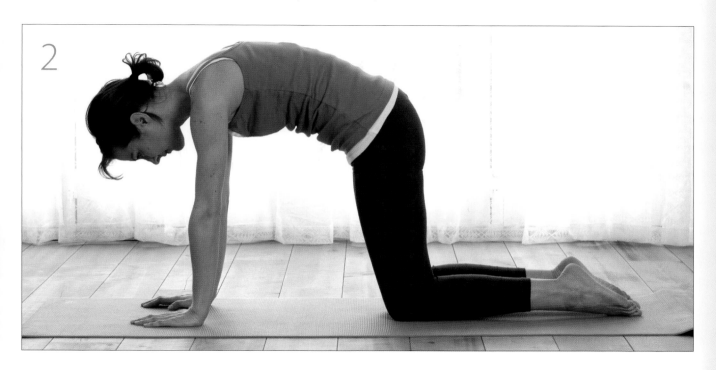

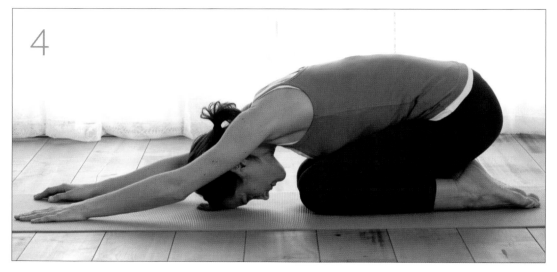

WATCH POINT
Try not to let your back sag because this could cause serious back injuries. You can avoid this by doing the stretch slowly and gently to make sure you are in control at all times.

back

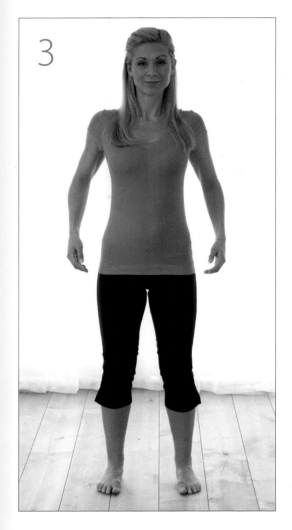

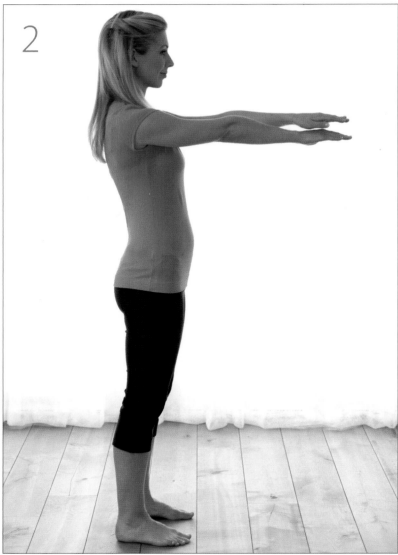

Shoulder rolls

This will ensure that you have fully warmed through the shoulders and chest and mobilized into the shoulder joints.

1 Stand with good posture and check that your feet are slightly wider than hip-width apart.

2 Make sure your knees are slightly bent and that your abdominal muscles are pulled in tight toward your spine.

3 Very slowly and gently, start to rotate through your shoulders by lifting your shoulders up, then behind. Each time, increase this movement and aim to make the circles bigger. Repeat the exercise ten times.

Arm swing

This will increase the flexibility of your chest muscles and help to loosen your upper back.

1 Stand with good posture, knees bent, and stomach pulled in. Lift both arms out to either side of your body.

2 In a slow and controlled manner, bring both arms in front so they cross over then back out to either side.

3 Be sure to keep your abdominal muscles pulled in to maintain good posture throughout. Repeat the exercise ten times.

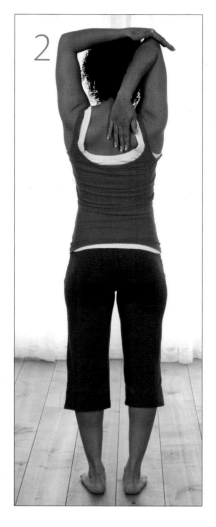 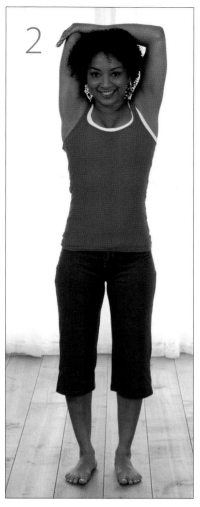 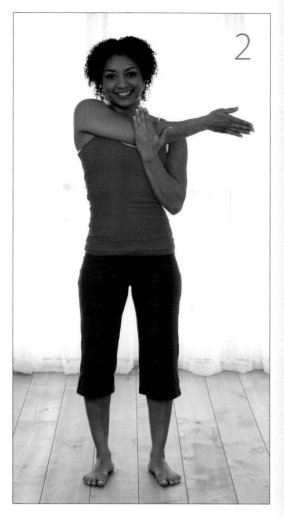

Triceps stretch

The muscle at the back of the upper arm is called the triceps. It is attached to the shoulder and the elbow and is activated by straightening the arm.

1 Stand with good posture, lift one arm above your head, and drop the palm of the hand behind the head between the shoulder blades.

2 Lift the other arm and support the stretching arm on the soft, fleshy part of the upper arm or just above the elbow. Hold this stretch on each arm for ten seconds.

Deltoid stretch

The muscles that form the shoulders are know as the deltoids and they are responsible for arm movement.

1 Stand with good posture, extend one arm out in front of you, and cross it in front of the midline of your body.

2 Keep both shoulders facing forward. Support the stretching arm on the fleshy part of the upper arm above the elbow. Hold this stretch on each arm for ten seconds.

THE BENEFITS OF STRETCHING
• It reduces the risk of injury during activity.
• It helps prevent post-exercise soreness.
• It improves your flexibility and range of movement.

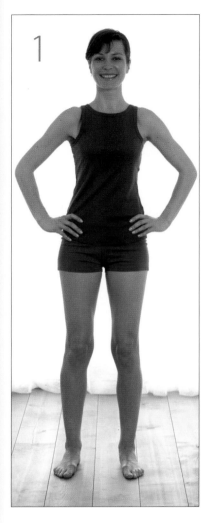
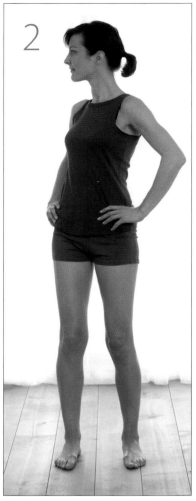
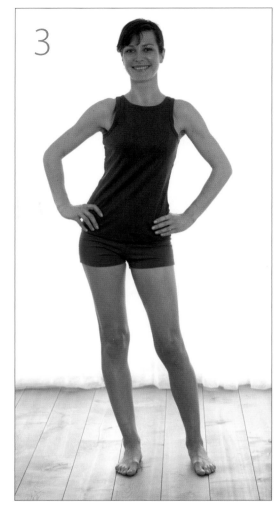

Waist twist

It's important not to move your hips and knees during this exercise, but move your arms like a hula dancer if it helps you to get into the right mood!

1 Stand up straight with your spine in neutral, and your knees slightly bent (soft, rather than "locked"). Keep your feet hip-width apart and your hands resting on your hips. Make sure your spine is in the neutral position.

2 Tighten your abdominal muscles by pulling your navel back toward your spine. Keeping your hips and knees still, rotate your shoulders and head to the right, then return to the center.

3 Now twist to the left, rotating your head and shoulders and keeping your hips and knees still.

4 Repeat this exercise a further five times on each side.

Hip circles

Try this exercise to warm up your pelvic muscles. Keep your torso still—only your pelvis should be moving during this exercise.

1 Stand up straight with your knees slightly bent, feet hip-width apart, and your hands resting lightly on your hips.

2 Gently draw in your navel toward your spine to tighten your abdominal muscles. Do not suck in your waist or hold your breath—this movement should feel light and subtle.

3 Slowly circle your pelvis to the right so that you are rotating in a full circle.

4 Repeat nine times to the right, then circle your hips ten times to the left.

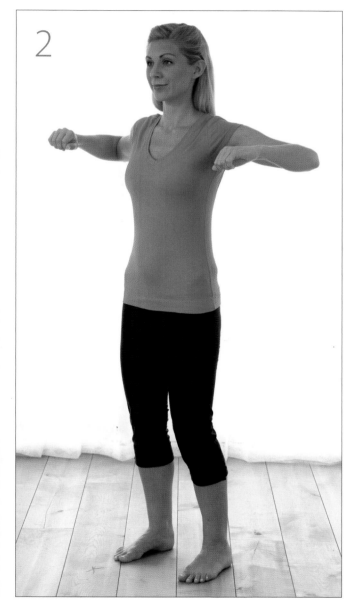

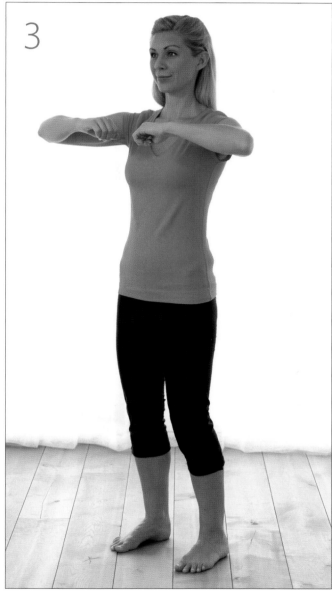

Easy chest stretch

This stretch targets the pectoral muscles, sometimes known as the "pecs," which are the major muscles at the front of the chest. It will also give your supraspinatus muscle, which runs along the top of your shoulder blades, a nice big stretch.

1 You can either stand with feet hip-width apart, or you can do this stretch while sitting on a chair. Whichever position you prefer, make sure that your back is straight and your head and neck are in line with your spine.

2 Bring your arms up to shoulder level and bend them at the elbows so that your hands are hovering in front of your chest. Make loose fists with your hands.

3 Leading from the elbow, gently rotate both arms backward so that you're squeezing your shoulder blades together. Your chest will automatically push out a little.

4 Hold for ten seconds, then release. Repeat this five times.

WATCH POINT
It's quite easy to get tired while doing this stretch but, if you persevere, you will soon feel the benefit of performing it correctly.

chest and shoulders

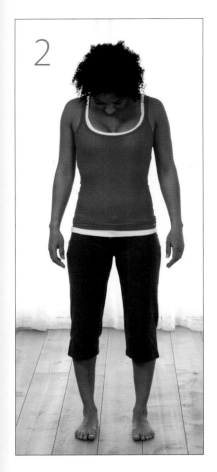

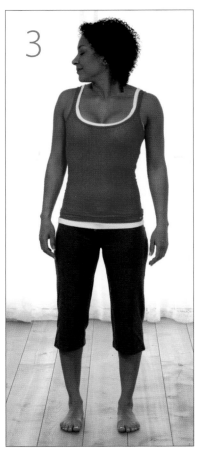

Neck stretches

This is a great substitute for a neck massage. It really helps to get your muscles loose, warm, and stretched. And it's much safer than rolling your neck, because it puts less of a strain on the surrounding muscles. Enure that your hips are facing forward at all times—only your head should move.

1 Stand up straight with feet hip-width apart. Relax your shoulders and look straight ahead.

2 Slowly lower your chin to your chest. Hold for a few seconds while you feel the stretch across the back of your neck and then gently raise your head so it's back in the starting position.

3 Next, rotate your head to the right and hold for a few seconds, then rotate your head to the left.

4 Hold for a few seconds, then return to the start position so you are looking straight ahead. Repeat the sequence three times.

Side bends

Do not do this exercise quickly with your arms above your head because this will make it hard to control the movement.

1 Stand up straight with your feet hip-width apart and your knees slightly bent, with your arms hanging loosely by your sides.

2 Tighten your abdominal muscles by gently pulling your navel toward your spine.

3 Keeping your back straight and without leaning forward, slowly bend to one side from the waist so that your hand slides down the side of your leg. Straighten up again.

4 Repeat on the other side. Repeat four more times on both sides.

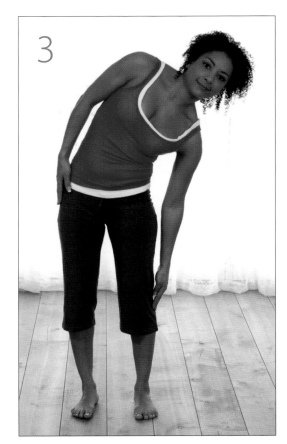

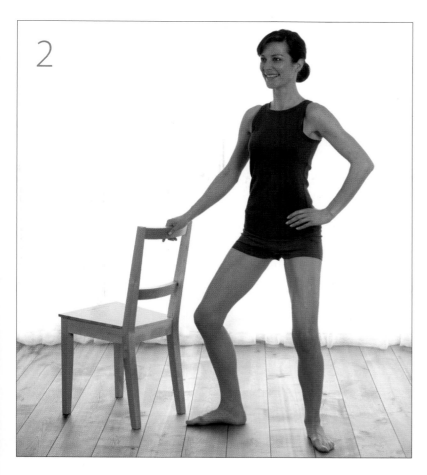

Knee bends

This exercise loosens the hip flexor muscles and helps to warm up all the leg muscles. Don't lock your knees as you do this, and bend only as far as is comfortable for you to go.

1 Stand with one hand resting on a support, such as a high-backed chair or a table, your feet hip-width apart and slightly turned out. Tighten your abdominal muscles.

2 Slowly bend your knees and lower your hips, then straighten up again. Use your buttock and leg muscles to lower and straighten. Repeat the exercise nine times.

WATCH POINT
Never point your toes inward while exercising—this can damage your knees.

Leg swings

This exercise warms up the hip joints. Don't swing your legs too high (about 45 degrees is high enough), and keep the movements controlled and flowing.

1 Stand with one hand resting on a support, such as a high-backed chair or a table, and balance on one leg with the knee slightly bent. Tighten your stomach muscles to protect your back.

2 Gently swing your other leg forward and backward. Keep your hips still as your leg moves from back to front.

3 Swing up to 20 times on one leg, then swap sides and swing on the other leg for the same duration.

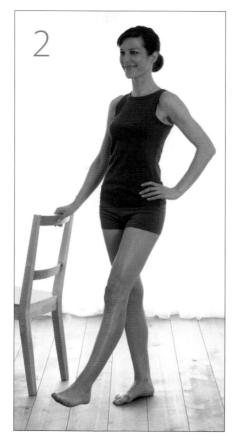

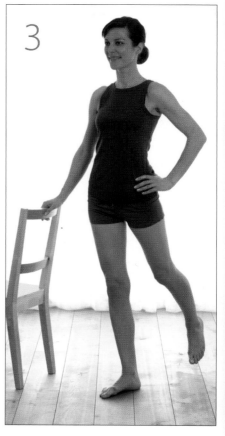

hips and legs

STANDING EXERCISES

The standing exercises in this section work the whole body. Some have traditional origins in exercise systems such as yoga and pilates. Make sure that all exercises are performed slowly, carefully, and with your full attention. You really do need to concentrate on what you're doing and think about how your body is responding to any exercise. If an action hurts or you do it quickly, then you are not performing it correctly. Movements should flow in a gentle, controlled manner. This enables your muscles to stretch naturally.

Shoulder press

This will help to tone through your shoulders and triceps as well as to promote good upper body posture and a balanced stance.

1 Stand with good posture, knees slightly bent, and stomach pulled in. Hold a weight in each hand at shoulder height.

2 With your palms facing forward and keeping your head level, press the weights overhead, extending your elbows.

3 Bring the weights together as you press them, hold for a second, then slowly lower to the start position. Repeat ten times.

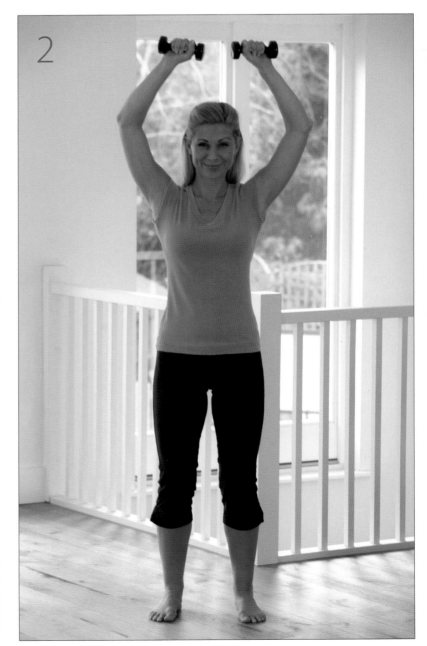

WATCH POINT
Keep your elbows slightly bent while performing this to avoid locking out your elbow joints.

Standing wall press-up

This exercise is a fantastic way to build upper body strength as well as tone through the back of your upper arm muscles and into your chest. If you keep your abdominal muscles pulled in, this exercise will also help to tone your stomach muscles.

1 Stand at arms' length away from a wall, with your feet shoulder-width apart. Place your hands against the wall, with your arms stretched out in front of you and your fingers pointing up.

2 Keeping your back straight and your head looking straight in front of you, slowly bend your arms at the elbows.

3 Aim to lower yourself a little way toward the wall and then push back to your start position. Repeat the exercise ten times.

WATCH POINT
If you want to increase the level of difficulty, try moving your legs farther back.

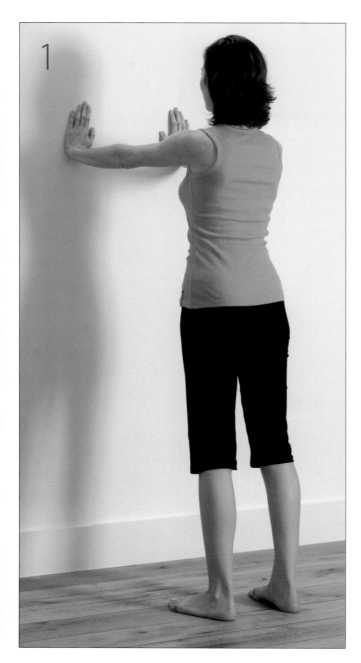

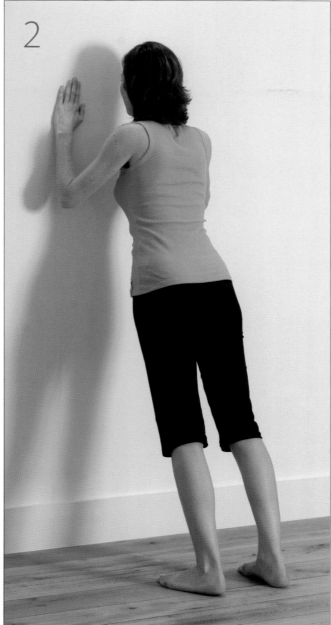

back and shoulders

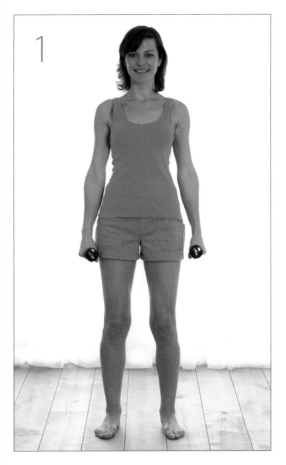

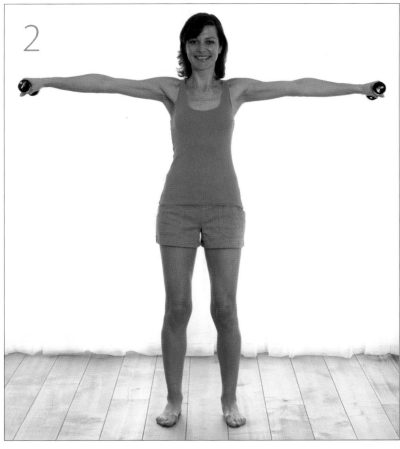

Side shoulder raise

This exercise will help to define your shoulders—it is also good for improving flexibility throughout your shoulder joints and will give you good posture.

1 Stand with your feet shoulder-width apart and your knees slightly bent. Hold the hand weights at your sides.

2 Slowly lift the weights out to the sides to shoulder level, keeping your elbows slightly bent. Keep your shoulders down and relaxed as you lift. If you find you are shrugging your shoulders up toward your ears, your weights may be too heavy.

3 Slowly lower the weights back to your start position. Repeat the exercise ten times.

SETTING THE PACE

It's important to work at the right intensity if you're toning up—put in too little effort and you won't notice much difference; throw yourself into the exercises and you may hurt yourself.

The aim of an exercise or toning program is to make your muscles work harder, either by increasing the number of repetitions of each exercise or by increasing the intensity of your workout. Your muscles will start to become tired during the last repetitions and you may feel a burning sensation in the area you're working but this is normal and will pass as soon as you rest.

Muscle soreness and stiffness is highly likely in the beginning, particularly if you're new to exercise, but if you can hardly move the next day, then you've overdone it. Rest up for a day or so and start again at a reduced intensity.

WATCH POINT
It's important to keep a slight bend in both arms as you lift them. Imagine both arms are pouring water from a kettle.

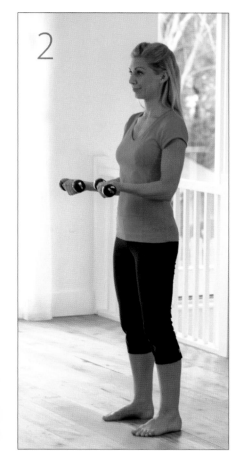

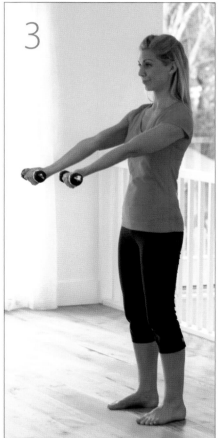

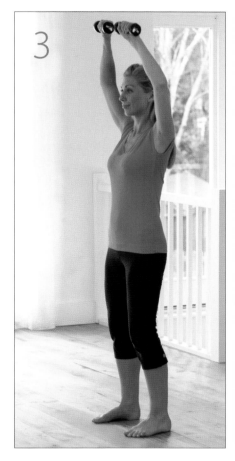

Turning press

This is a great time-saving exercise, as it targets several upper body muscles at once, including your triceps, biceps, and shoulders.

1 Stand with your feet hip-width apart, upper body straight, knees soft, and stomach pulled in.

2 Hold a weight in each hand with the palms facing directly in front of your shoulders with your elbows bent.

3 In one continuous flowing movement, straighten the elbows and lift the weights overhead, twisting the hands until the palms face out. Lower your arms and twist your palms to face in again. Repeat the exercise ten times.

Front raises

This simple exercise is designed to sculpt your shoulders and create tone and definition through the front of your arms.

1 Stand with good posture, your feet hip-width apart, and knees soft. Keep your abdominal muscles tight and chest relaxed.

2 Hold a weight in each hand with palms facing in, weights hanging loosely by your thighs.

3 In a slow and controlled smooth move, lift both arms up forward and straight to shoulder height, then slowly lower both arms back to the start position. Repeat ten times.

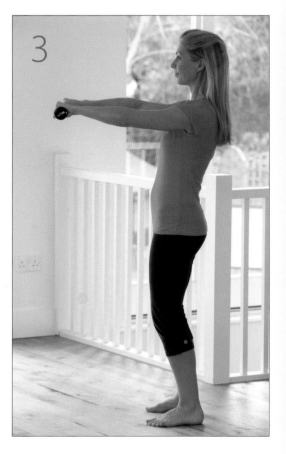

shoulders and arms

Reach and squat using an exercise ball

It is important to warm up before any exercise. In addition to your usual stretching routine, it is a good idea to perform this exercise before attempting other exercises using a ball. It will help to mobilize your body and focus your mind.

1 Stand tall with your feet wide apart, holding the ball above your head.

2 Bend your knees and, keeping your back straight, bring the ball toward the floor.

3 Straighten your knees and reach up again. Repeat four or five times.

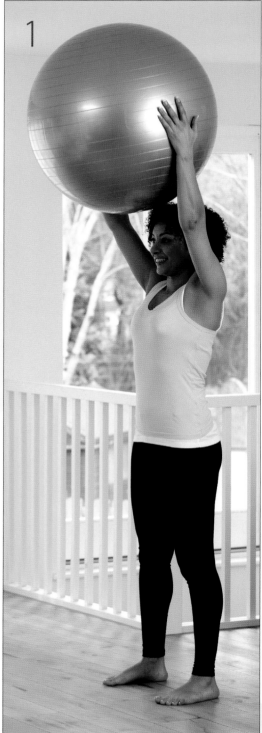

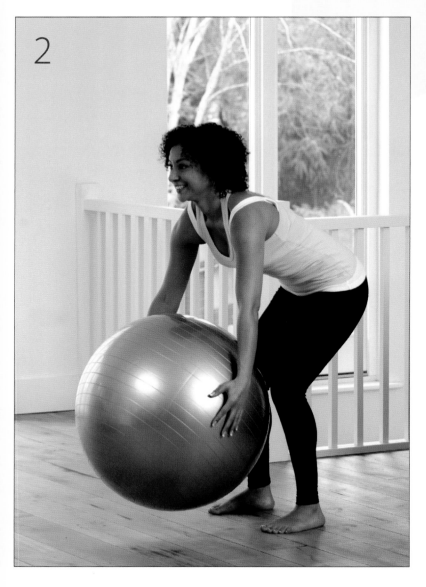

Double shoulder stretch using an exercise ball

This exercise works the muscles at the back and the sides of the neck which lift the shoulders. It will improve flexibility in your shoulders and release tension in your chest muscles.

1 Stand with the ball at chest height between you and the wall. Your hands should be on the ball and your arms slightly bent. Keep your feet hip-width apart.

2 Tighten your abdominal muscles and concentrate on keeping your spine properly aligned.

3 Push the ball up the wall until your biceps are level with your ears. Hold for a count of five, then return to the starting position. Repeat four or five times.

WATCH POINT

If you are too close to the wall, you will not feel the stretch. If you are too far away from the wall, your back will arch and your heels will come off the ground. Avoid this exercise if you experience any shoulder or neck pain.

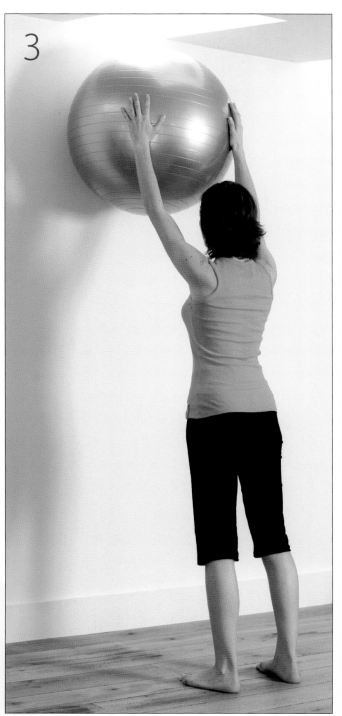

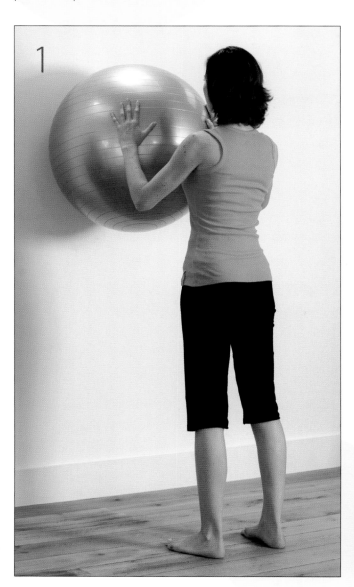

shoulders

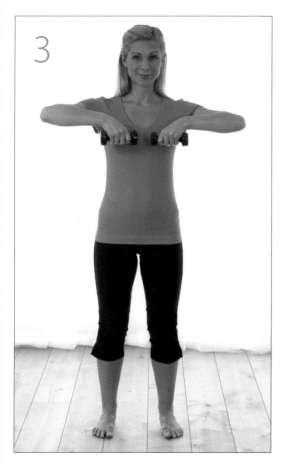 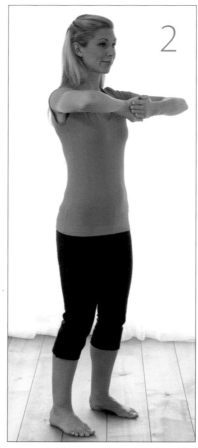 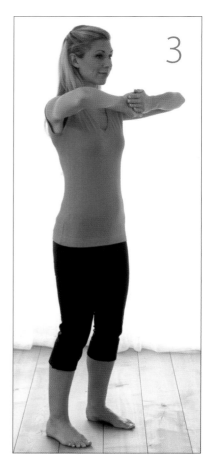

Upright pull

This exercise focuses on toning through your shoulders, biceps, and back, which will help you achieve a beautifully toned upper body.

1 Stand with your feet shoulder-width apart and your knees slightly bent.

2 Hold a weight in each hand, side by side at thigh level, keeping your palms facing toward your thighs.

3 Slowly bring the weights up toward your collarbone, until your elbows are about shoulder height. Keep your shoulders down and relaxed as you lift. If you find you are shrugging your shoulders up toward your ears, your weights may be too heavy.

4 Slowly lower the weights to the start position. Repeat the exercise ten times.

Bust lift

This exercise targets the chest muscle which is responsible for supporting the bust. If this muscle is not exercised, it will become less supportive, which means the bust begins to droop. This is a great way of toning and giving yourself a bust lift.

1 Stand upright with good posture, knees slightly bent, feet hip-width distance apart, and stomach pulled in toward your spine.

2 Extend your arms out in front of you at chest height, bend the elbows and join the hands by the palms facing into each other.

3 Stay in this position, press into your palms and, holding this squeeze, slowly lift your palms a little bit higher. Hold for a second while still applying the squeeze, then slowly lower to the start position, release the squeeze for a second, then re-apply and lift. Repeat ten times.

WATCH POINT
Keep this very slow and controlled. The more pressure you apply through the squeeze, the harder you work on lifting the bust.

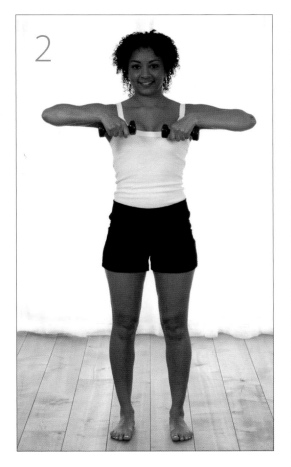

Chest press

This exercise targets two muscles—your triceps and your chest muscle. This is a great exercise for women, as it tightens the muscles that support your bust, giving you a good bust lift.

1 Stand with a good upright posture, knees soft and your feet hip-width apart.

2 Using a weight in each hand, bend your arms so your hands are in front of your shoulders.

3 Gently extend your arms straight out, keeping them at shoulder height.

4 Hold for a second when your arms are fully extended. Slowly return your arms to the start position. Repeat the exercise ten times.

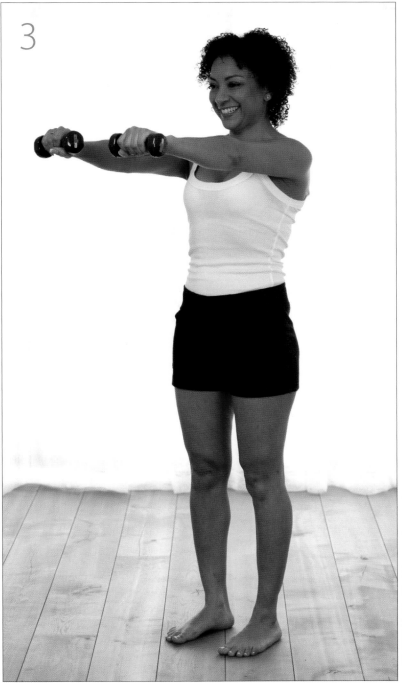

WATCH POINT
Focus on engaging your abdominal muscles, by pulling your navel tight to your spine. This helps to protect your back.

chest and arms

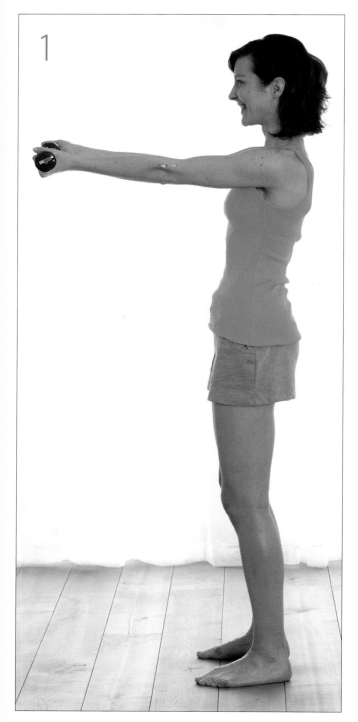

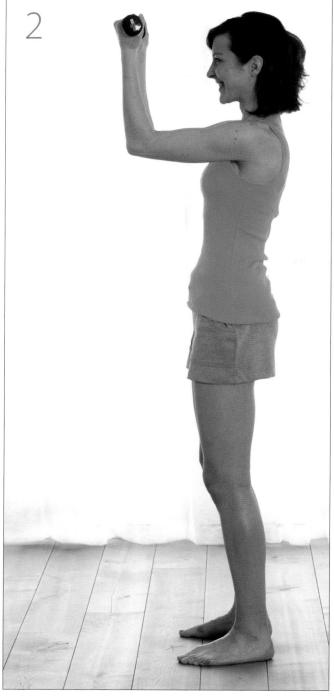

Bicep curl

The biceps are the muscles at the front of the upper arms. They are relatively easy to tone, so practicing this exercise will help to give you shapely arms that you'll want to show off.

1 Stand up tall with feet hip-width apart and knees soft. Extend your arms out in front of you with palms facing upward, holding a dumbbell in each hand.

2 Bend your elbows and bring both your hands in toward your shoulders so that your arms form right-angles.

3 Reverse the movement so that your elbows are fully extended in front of you again. Keep your elbows soft at all times during the in and out movement. Repeat the movement ten times.

arms

Arm circles

This easy-to-follow exercise will improve mobility and definition in your shoulders. You can increase the intensity by using hand weights or by simply creating bigger circles.

1 Stand straight with your feet shoulder-width apart. Your arms should be straight out to the sides so that your body forms a T-shape.

2 Starting slowly, make small, circular motions with both arms moving in the same direction.

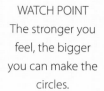

WATCH POINT
The stronger you feel, the bigger you can make the circles.

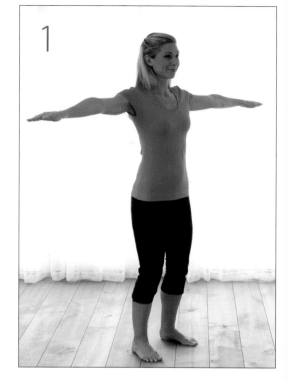

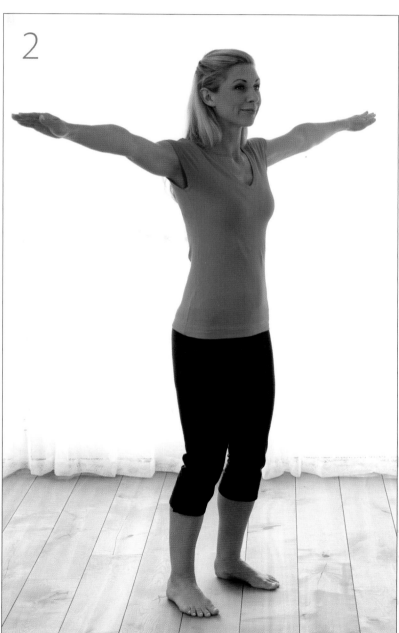

3 Focus on keeping your knees soft and your abdominal muscles pulled in throughout. Perform ten circles, then return to the starting position.

4 Repeat the exercise ten times, but this time making circles in the opposite direction.

shoulders and arms

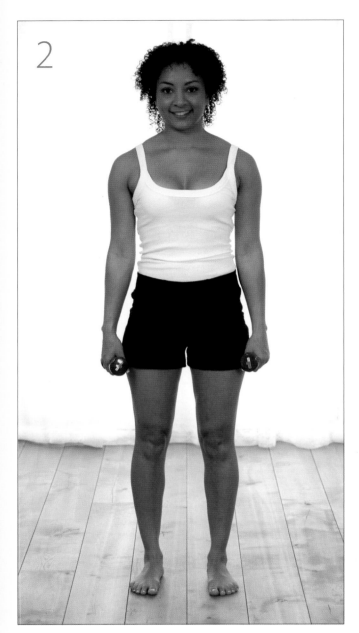

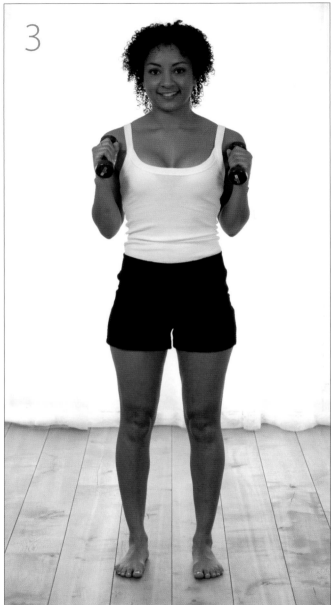

Front arm toner

Also known as the hammer curl, this exercise tones through the front of your upper arms and also works on strengthening your forearm muscles.

1 Stand with your feet shoulder-width apart, knees soft, elbows fixed, and stomach pulled in tight to promote good upper body posture.

2 With a weight in each hand, let both arms hang down long by the side of your body, fully straightened with your palms facing in toward your body.

3 Simultaneously lift your weights upward, without moving your elbows, hold for a second, then slowly lower back to your start position. Repeat the lift ten times.

arms

Arm opener

This exercise works by toning the biceps in your front upper arms. The exercise will firm the biceps, not bulk them out.

1 Stand with your feet shoulder-width apart, knees soft, elbows fixed, and stomach pulled in tight to promote good upper body posture.

2 Have your arms by your side with your elbows bent and your arms in an L-shape, a weight in each hand.

3 With your palms facing in toward each other, slowly open your forearms out to either side, while still keeping your elbows tucked into your sides. Hold for a second, then slowly return to a start position. Repeat ten times.

WATCH POINT
Keep this exercise slow and controlled. It is important to keep your elbows locked in tight to your sides.

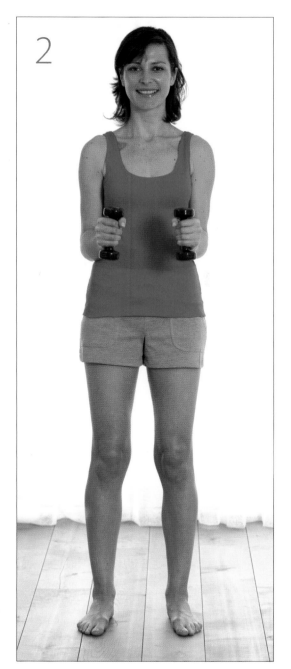

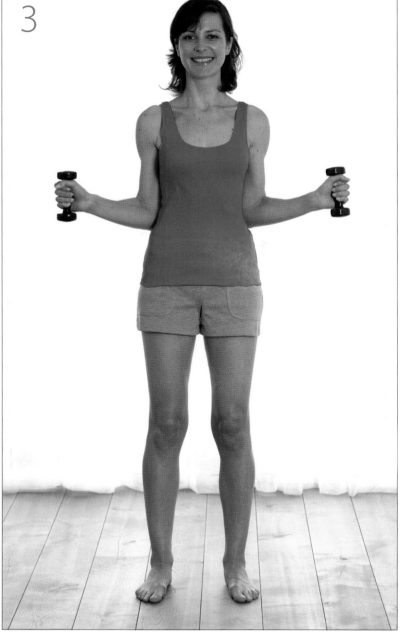

arms

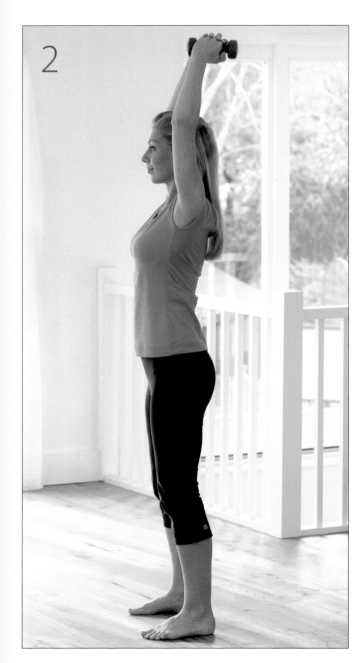
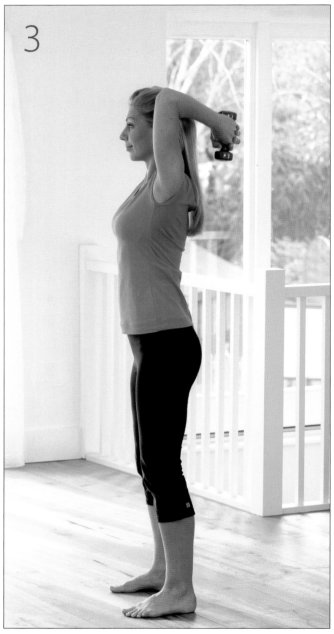

Triceps extension

The triceps are the muscles at the back of the upper arms. If they're left to go slack, it can lead to the dreaded "flabby arm" effect, where loose skin on the underside of your arm wobbles as you wave. It's classically a hard muscle to target, but this exercise will help to tighten and tone them.

1 Stand with feet hip-width apart. Pick up a heavy object with both hands—choose something that you can work comfortably with, such as a dumbbell or a heavy book.

2 Bring the object over your head keeping your arms straight as you do this.

3 Bend your arms at the elbows, so you slowly lower it down between your shoulder blades.

4 Reverse the movement by straightening your arms so you bring the object directly back above your head. Do this slowly, so you're in control of the movement. Repeat the movement ten times.

WATCH POINT
Choose a weight that's challenging but not so heavy that you can't control it—you don't want to end up dropping it on your head.

arms

Triceps kick-back

This exercise isolates the back of the upper arm, specifically targeting the troublesome area sometimes referred to as "auntie's arms." Always ensure you use a sturdy chair.

1 Kneel over a chair, with one arm supporting your body and one knee bent on the chair. Ensure that the elbow of the supporting arm stays soft and that the knee of the leg extended to the floor is also soft.

2 With your weight in one hand, position your upper arm so it is parallel to the floor and bent at the elbow.

3 Slowly extend the arm until it is straight, then slowly return and repeat. Perform ten repetitions on one arm and then repeat on the other arm, by turning around and placing your opposite leg on the chair.

WATCH POINT
For a greater range of motion, the upper arm can be positioned with the elbow at a slightly higher angle than the shoulder.

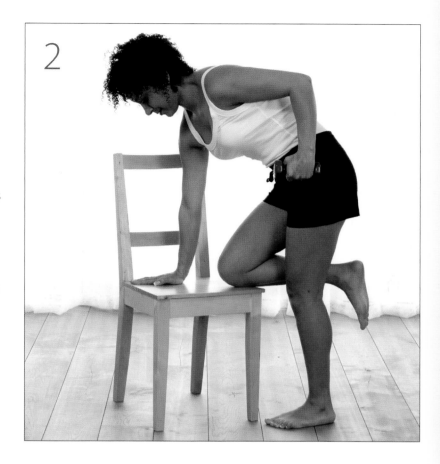

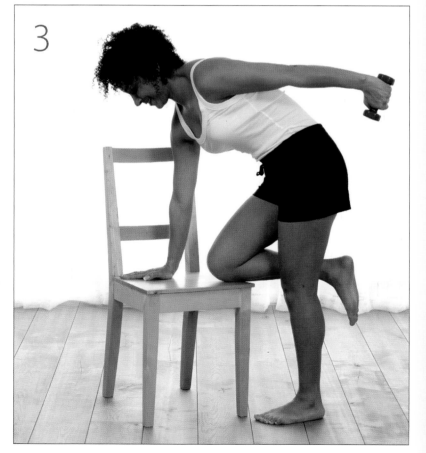

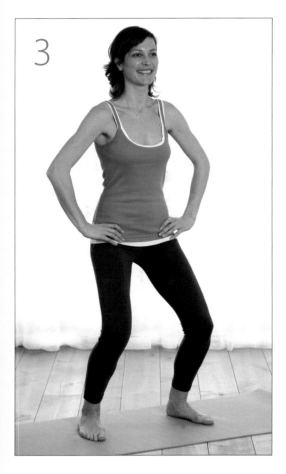

Basic squat

If you only ever do one type of hip and thigh exercise, make it a squat, which really hits the spot! Targeting the buttocks and tops of the thighs, this easy exercise is great for toning up those trouble spots. Remember to keep your knees soft (slightly bent) throughout.

1 Stand up with good posture, your feet hip-width apart, and your hands on your hips.

2 Tighten your abdominal muscles by gently pulling your navel toward your spine.

3 Bend your knees and squat as if you were going to sit down. Only squat as far as is comfortable and without losing your balance.

4 Return to the standing position by pushing through your heels, keeping your knees slightly bent as you do so. Repeat the exercise ten times.

WATCH POINT
Squats work the hip extensors, hamstrings (back of thigh muscles), and quadriceps (front of thigh muscles). Tight quads and hamstrings cause poor posture and lower back pain so it's very important to keep them in good working order.

Wide squat

Wide squats are great for toning your inner thigh muscles and the front and back of the thighs. Try not to wobble.

1 Stand up with good posture, your feet wide apart and your toes turned out. Keep your hands on your hips.

2 Tighten your abdominal muscles by gently pulling your navel toward your spine.

3 Bend your knees and lower your bottom as if you were going to sit down on a low chair.

4 Go as low as you can without wobbling forward. Return to a standing position by pushing through your heels, keeping your knees slightly bent as you do so. Repeat ten times.

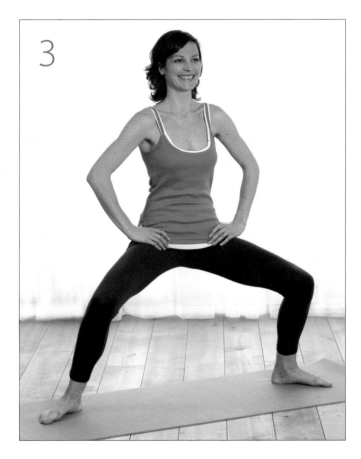

thighs and hips

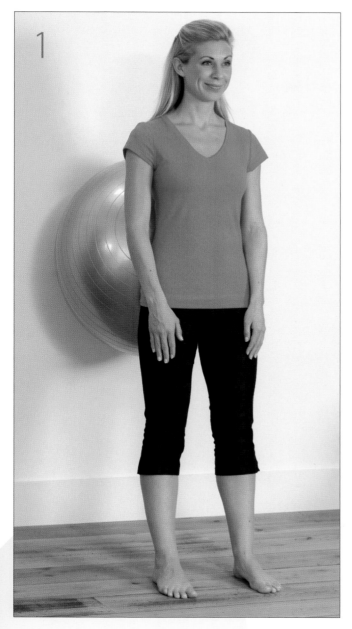

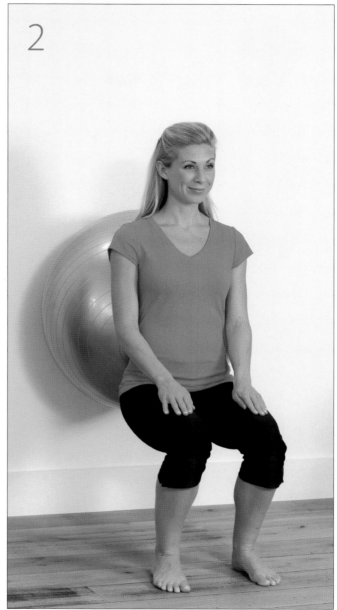

Squat—variation using an exercise ball

Don't use a mat for this exercise because of the risk of slipping.

1 Stand with the ball between your lower back and the wall and your feet hip-width apart. Rest your hands on your thighs and tighten your abdominal muscles.

2 Roll down to a seated squat position until your thighs are horizontal. Hold for a count of five, then slowly stand up. Repeat the movement ten times.

3 To make this more challenging, hold weights by your side to further load the quadriceps.

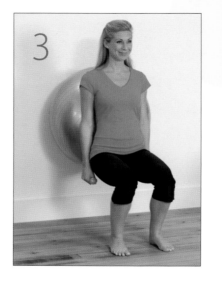

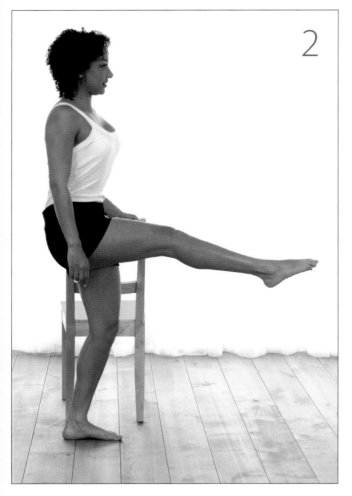

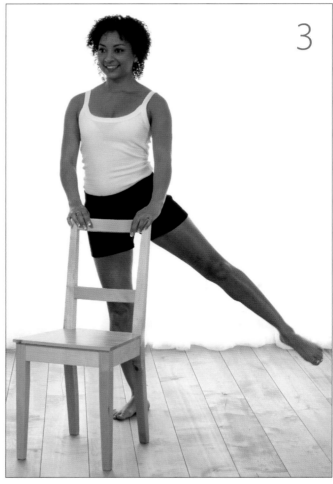

Front leg raise

This exercise strengthens and tones the front of your thighs (quadriceps) and increases your hip flexibility.

1 Stand up straight with your feet together and hold on to the back of a chair turned sideways with your left hand to balance. Tighten your stomach muscles.

2 With your left leg slightly bent, raise your right leg out in front of you as far as is comfortable. Hold for a count of three.

3 Lower your leg. Perform ten repetitions on that leg, then repeat on the other leg.

WATCH POINT
Keep your body straight and both knees soft throughout.

Lateral leg raise

This exercise helps to tone and tighten your outer thigh muscles and your hips, as well as improve your balance.

1 Stand up straight with good posture, hands by your sides and feet together, holding on to the back of a chair with both hands to maintain your balance.

2 Tighten your abdominal muscles by gently drawing in your navel toward your spine. This will protect your lower back muscles during the exercise.

3 Raise one leg out to the side at an angle of about 45 degrees. Keep your toes pointing forward and hold for a count of three, then relax. Perform ten repetitions on one leg, then repeat using the other leg.

thighs and hips

3

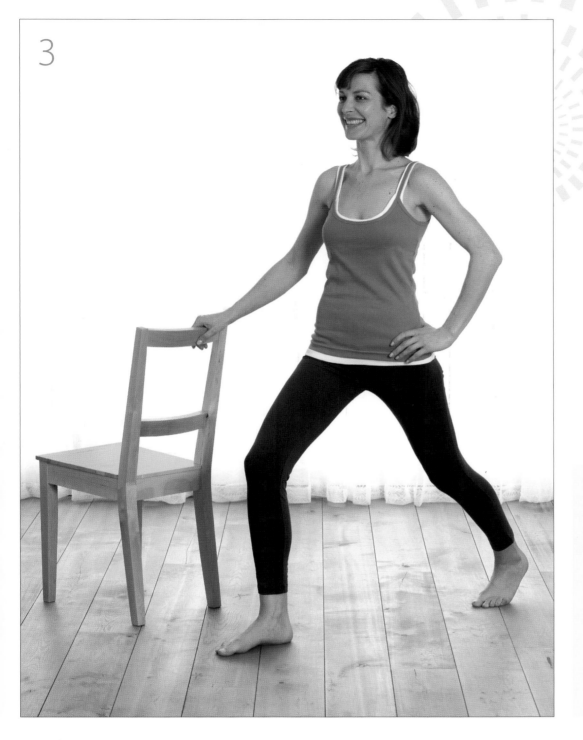

WATCH POINT
For best results, keep your buttocks tensed throughout. It's harder but better for you in the long run. Keep movements smooth and fluid and move only as far as is comfortable.

Rear leg raise

This strengthens and tones the buttocks, lower back, back of the hips, and hamstrings. It also helps with your balance.

1 Stand up straight with your feet together and use your right hand to hold on to the back of a chair turned sideways to help maintain your balance.

2 Pull in your stomach muscles to support your back and tighten your buttock muscles.

3 Stretch your left leg back, and touch the floor with your toes. Hold this position for a count of three, then return to the start. Perform ten repetitions on one leg, then repeat on the other leg.

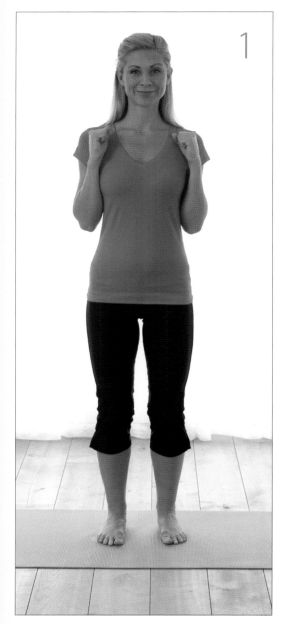

1

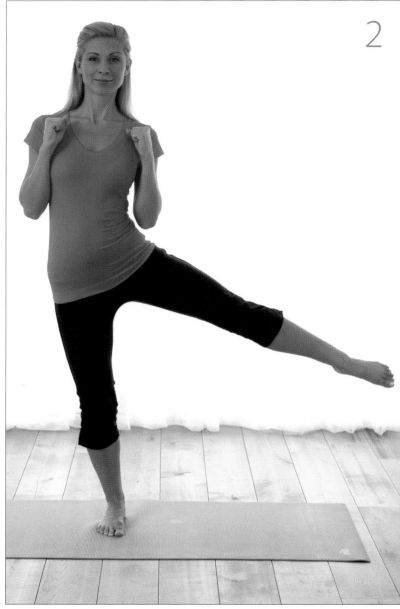

2

Side kick

The side kick is an energetic exercise that will get your heart rate pumping and really burn some calories. It's great for toning the hamstrings and quads and it will give your waist a workout too.

1 Stand with feet hip-width apart. Bring your hands up to your chest and form loose fists, while keeping your elbows bent and by your sides to help you balance.

2 Raise your left leg off the floor and kick it out to the side in a swift, controlled move. Be careful not to flick your leg, as you could jar your knee or hip if you do so.

3 Bring your leg back to the starting position and repeat the movement ten times.

4 Return to starting position and repeat the movement ten times with your right leg.

WATCH POINT
Be careful that you don't use too much force to shoot your leg out to the side or you may end up straining a muscle or jarring your knee.

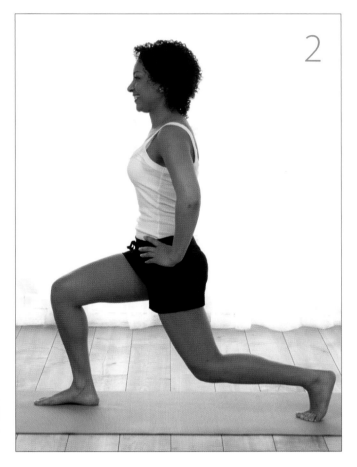

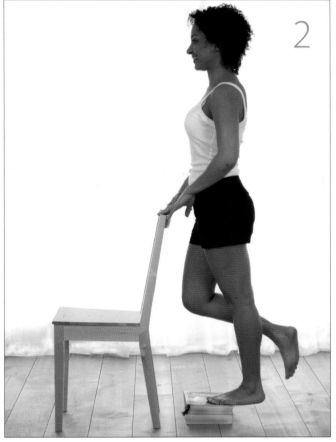

Lunge

Lunging is great for strengthening and toning the muscles in the buttocks and is a firm favorite among personal fitness trainers.

1 Stand with feet hip-width apart. Rest your hands on your hips or by your sides.

2 Step forward with your right leg, bending your knee so your thigh is almost at a right-angle to the floor. Your right foot should be flat on the floor. Your left leg should be slightly bent at the knee and the ball of your left foot should be resting on the floor behind you, with your heel slightly in the air.

3 Hold for a second, then push off the floor with your right foot and return to the starting position. Repeat the movement with alternate legs. Aim to do around five lunges on each side.

WATCH POINT
Don't rush the lunge or go down too far or you'll end up banging your knee on the floor.

Standing calf raises

Calf muscles are hard to target, although studies have shown that walking in high heels can help to tone them up! For really shapely calves, we recommend you try this exercise instead.

1 Stand with both feet near the edge of a raised object such as a stair or a big chunky book. Place the ball of your left foot on the edge of the object, letting your heel extend off the edge.

2 Hold on to a wall or a chair for support and, lifting your right leg into the air slightly by bending at the knee, gently let your left heel drop down until you feel the stretch in your calf. Carefully control the move: keep your back straight, your head up, and your left leg straight.

3 Rise up on to your left toe as high as you can and hold for a second while flexing the calf muscle.

4 Carefully return to the starting position, then repeat with the right leg. Aim to do ten repetitions on each foot, but do not do more than is comfortable for you. If this is a new exercise to you, begin with fewer repetitions.

SEATED EXERCISES

Even if you're office-bound for a large part of the day or spend a lot of time traveling, you can still sneak in a few exercises while you are sitting down to keep your posture aligned and your muscles toned. You'll need a straight-backed, sturdy chair for these exercises—not one on casters.

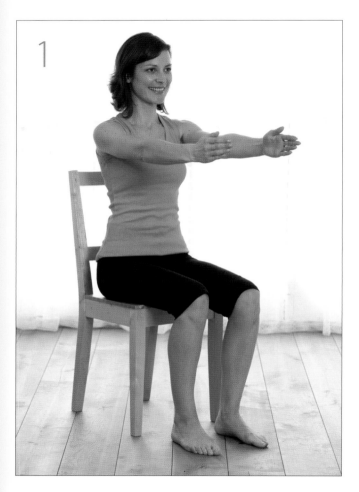

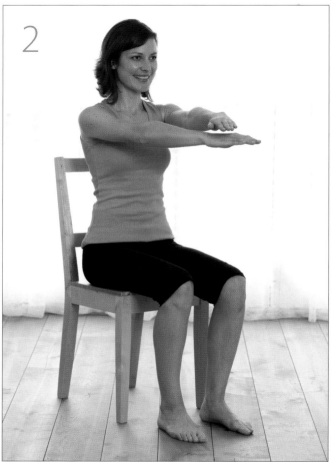

Criss-cross arms

This simple exercise tones your triceps, biceps, and chest muscles.

1 Sit with good posture, arms extended out in front of you, palms facing each other.

2 Cross your left arm over the right, turning your palms down along the way. Pause, then return to the starting position.

3 Perform ten repetitions for one arm and then repeat the same number on the other arm.

WATCH POINT
Focus on keeping your abdominal muscles pulled in throughout. To make this more of a challenge, try holding weights.

Bent-over arm shaper

This seated exercise will target your arms and your upper back muscles and improve your upper body flexibility and posture.

1 Holding a weight in each hand, sit on the edge of your chair, leaning forward, with arms hanging down, feet slightly apart.

2 Keep your abdominal muscles pulled in to stop you collapsing your back onto your legs.

3 Lift your arms out to the sides, up to shoulder level, squeezing your shoulder blades together.

4 Keep the elbows slightly bent and only lift to your shoulders. Lower the arms and repeat the exercise ten times.

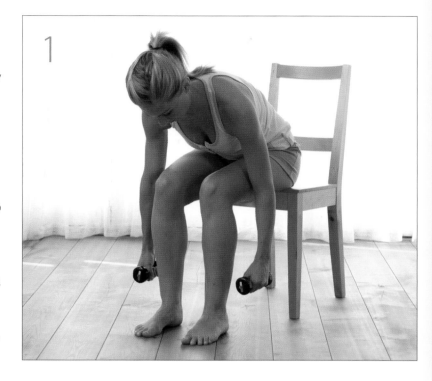

WATCH POINT
To make sure you keep your arms slightly bent, imagine you are pouring water from a kettle.

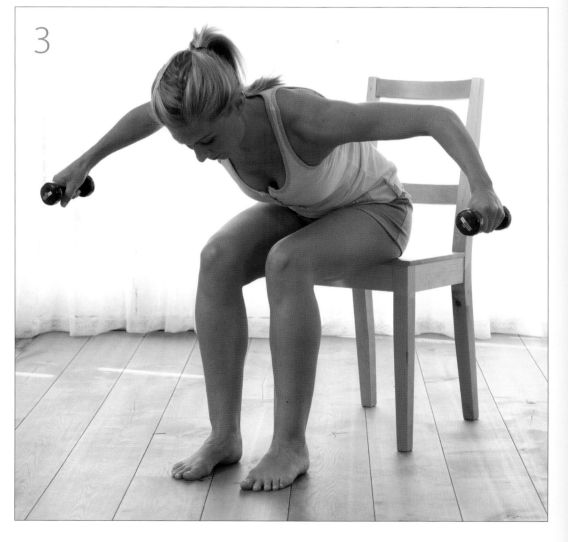

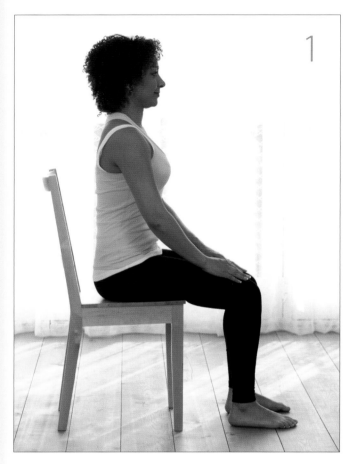

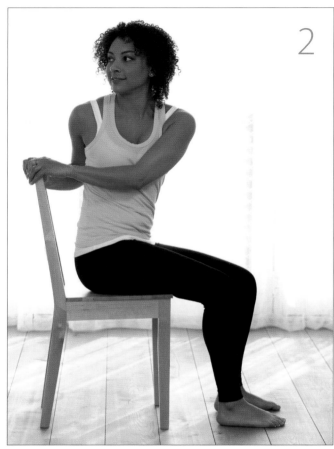

Spine rotation

This exercise gently mobilizes your spine. It is a useful exercise to include in your workout as it prepares the spine for other more challenging exercises.

1 Sit forward on a chair with your back straight and your hands resting on your thighs. Your knees should be over your ankles.

2 Tighten your abdominal muscles. Keeping your hips and knees forward, slowly rotate your upper body to the right until you can put both hands on the back of the chair.

3 Hold for a count of ten, then return to the center. Repeat the exercise, twisting to the left. Perform ten reps on each side.

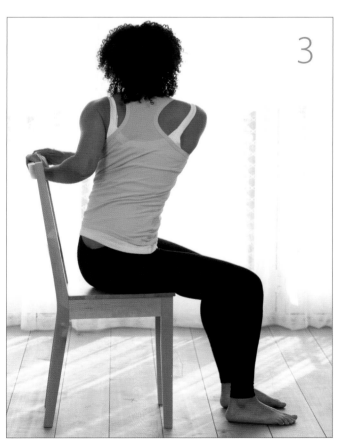

Seated reverse abdominal curl

This is an easy exercise that can be done almost anywhere. It works your rectus abdominis abdominal muscles. Try to avoid sagging or arching the back and hold your abdominal muscles in tight throughout the movement.

1 Sit on a stool or on a bench with your spine in neutral. Set your abdominal muscles to tighten them and extend your arms in front of you at shoulder height.

2 Slowly lean your torso and shoulders backward, keeping the spine rigid, as far back as is comfortable.

3 Hold the position for a count of two, then return to the starting position. Perform ten repetitions.

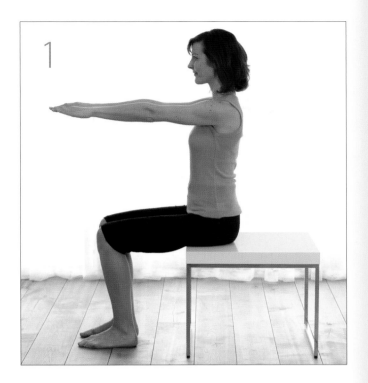

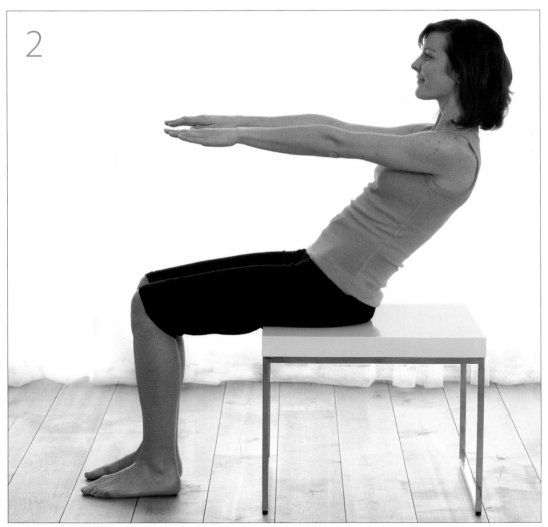

stomach

Seated knee lift

This seated exercise will work your rectus abdominis—the muscle that runs down the front of your stomach. Make sure your movements are controlled and flowing.

1 Sit on the edge of a chair with your knees bent and pressed together and your feet flat on the floor. Hold on to the sides of the chair, then tighten your stomach muscles.

2 Lean back slightly and lift your feet a few inches off the ground, keeping your knees bent and pressed together.

3 Slowly pull your knees in toward your chest and curl your upper body forward. Then lower your feet to the floor. Rest for a count of three. Aim to perform ten repetitions.

WATCH POINT
Don't lean too far forward or you'll fall off the chair!

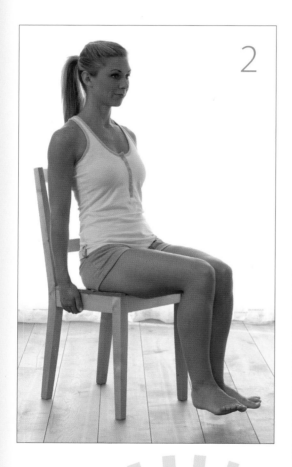

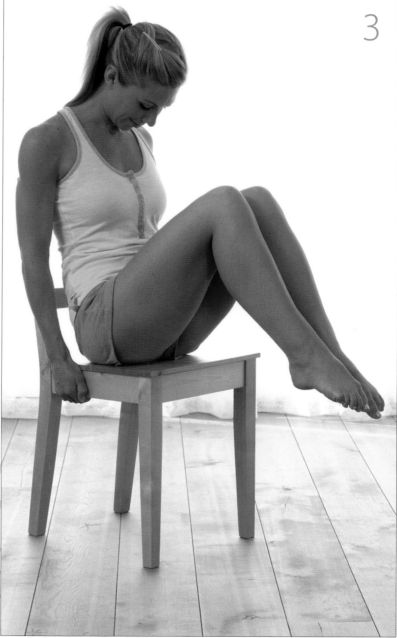

stomach

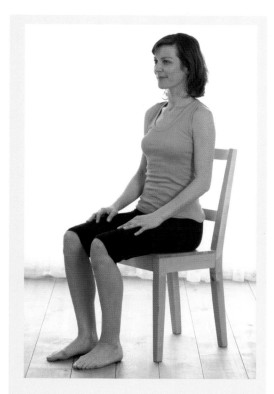

SITTING PRETTY

If you sit properly, not only will those extra inches of stomach appear to diminish but you'll be doing your back a favor, too!

Sit up straight with both feet on the floor, hip-width apart, and with your knees directly over your feet (don't tuck your feet under the chair).

Try not to slump backward or forward because you'll put pressure on your lower back. Avoid crossing your legs, because this pushes your spine out of alignment.

Tighten your abdominal muscles by gently pulling in your navel toward your backbone. Relax your shoulders and gently squeeze your shoulder blades together to stop them from rounding.

Make this position second nature and you'll soon notice the difference—you'll be able to breathe more deeply because your abdomen won't be squashed.

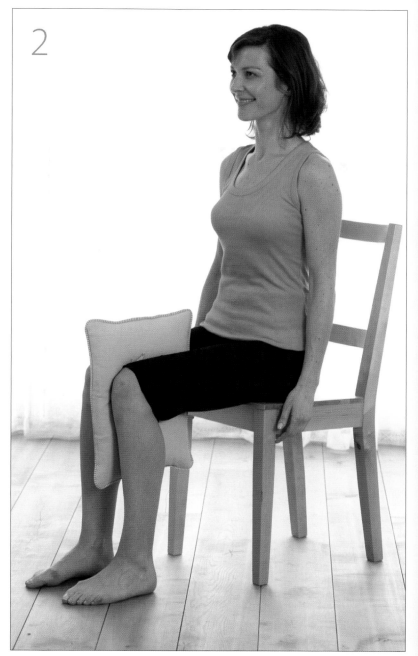

Simple seated thigh squeeze

This tones and strengthens your inner thighs. Make this exercise harder by increasing the time of the squeeze and by using something with more resistance, such as a semi-inflated ball.

1 Sit up straight on a chair with your knees bent and feet together.

2 Place a cushion between your thighs. Squeeze the cushion as hard as possible for a count of five, then release. Repeat the exercise ten times.

Seated leg extension

This easy exercise is great for toning the quadriceps, the muscles at the front of your thighs.

1 Sit up straight with good posture. Tighten your abdominal muscles by pulling in your navel toward your spine—this will protect your back muscles during this exercise.

2 Press your knees together and straighten one leg. Hold and release. Perform ten repetitions for one leg, then repeat for the other leg.

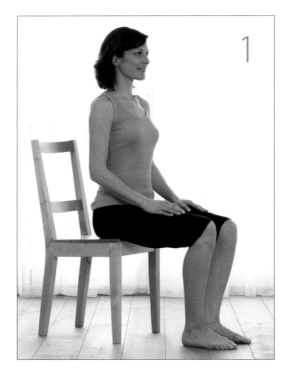

WATCH POINT
To make this more effective, you can use ankle weights to strengthen the intensity of the exercise.

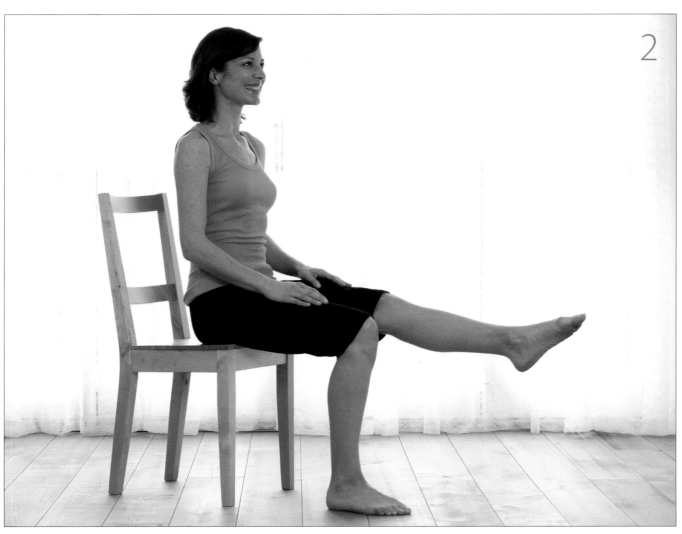

thighs and hips

Sitting properly using an exercise ball

Exercises with a ball require you to keep your spine in neutral. This means that you maintain the natural curve in your back (see posture, page 11), and avoid arching your back or pressing it so far down that you lose its natural curve.

1 Sit on the ball with your back straight and both feet placed on the floor, hip-width apart. Set your abdominal muscles (see box below).

2 Relax your shoulders and gently squeeze your shoulder blades together to stop them from becoming rounded. If you force your shoulders back and your lower back arches away from the ball, your shoulders are still too rounded.

3 Try to think of your head sitting naturally on your shoulders, neither pulling it forward nor pushing it back. Keep your breathing slow and steady as you maintain a balaced posture.

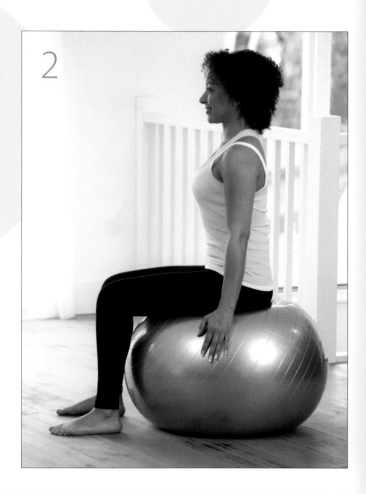

HOW TO SET YOUR ABDOMINAL MUSCLES

When you work out on the ball, you are constantly switching on your core muscles to keep your back and the ball still, so correct technique is vital. You have to set your abdominals in nearly every exercise, and practicing the setting action is a very important preliminary step.

Sit comfortably on the center of the ball and place one hand behind you in the small of your back.

Now place your other hand on your lower abdomen, below your navel. The deep abdominals lie beneath this area. Lengthen your spine but relax your shoulders and your breathing.

Imagine a belt under your hands. Gently draw your front hand toward your back as though tightening the belt one notch.

This setting action should feel light and subtle. If you suck in your waist or hold your breath, the action becomes ineffective as you won't be reaching the deep stabilizing muscles.

stomach

Sitting balance using an exercise ball

Sitting on the ball and lifting your feet from the floor is a great way to train your core stabilizing muscles.

1 Sit on the ball with your feet hip-width apart.

2 Lift one foot off the floor and hold it there for a count of five.

3 Put the foot down, then lift the other foot. Repeat ten times on each side.

WATCH POINT
If you lift your feet too high, you will wobble on the ball and lose your postural alignment.

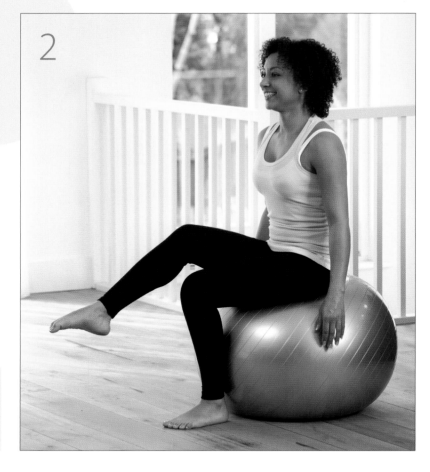

Toe taps using an exercise ball

This exercise helps to tone and stretch your legs and can also be used as a gentle warm-up for more difficult exercises.

1 Sit on the ball with your feet hip-width apart and flat on the floor, your arms hanging loosely by your sides.

2 Stretching out one leg, tap the toes of one foot on the floor in front of you ten times.

3 Return to the starting position and repeat on the other side.

stomach

Hip circles using an exercise ball

This exercise promotes strength and mobility in your spine and stabilizing pelvic muscles. Tighten your abdominal muscles throughout the exercise.

1 Sit on the ball with your feet shoulder-width apart and your hands touching the ball on either side.

2 Tighten your abdominal muscles and use your pelvis to rotate the ball slowly three times to the right in small clockwise circles.

3 Repeat on the other side—working counterclockwise.

WATCH POINT
Adding arm or leg movements will challenge your balance and coordination and increase the intensity of the exercise.

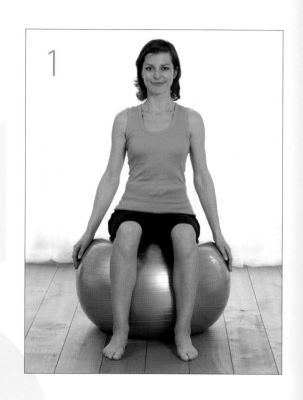

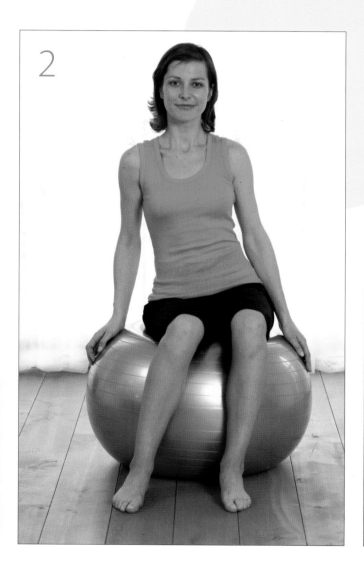

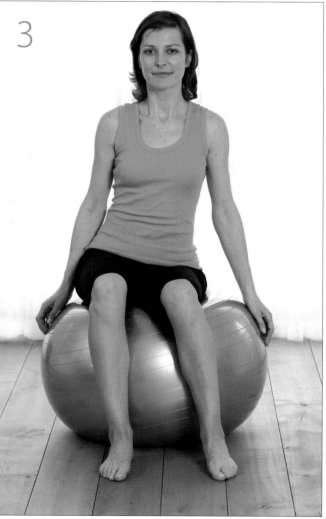

stomach

FLOOR EXERCISES

This section has a range of floor exercises designed to develop strength and flexibility and improve core stability. Don't worry if you can't complete the full range of movement suggested in each exercise—as you get fitter this will become easier. Include some floor exercises in your regular workout sessions and you will soon notice how your body feels more toned and looks trimmer.

WATCH POINT
Engage your stomach muscles to keep your back straight and avoid risk of injury.

Press-ups

This is a good all-round exercise for toning the major muscles in the arms. It's really good for developing upper-body strength and balancing out a pear-shaped figure.

1 Lie face-down on the floor, with your forehead resting on the backs of your hands. Slide your hands around to rest at shoulder level and try to find your ideal "press-up" position either side of your chest.

2 Use your arms to lift your upper body off the floor and bring your knees in toward your chest a little so they're resting on the floor, taking most of your body weight. Cross your feet at the ankles and raise them off the floor slightly. This should automatically cause your body weight to shift forward on to your arms and hands.

3 Bend your elbows and gently lower your upper body back down to the floor, keeping your head and shoulders level and in line with your spine at all times. Then push off the floor with your hands, raising your upper body into the air. Aim to get your arms straight, while keeping your elbows soft. Repeat this movement. Try to do two sets of ten repetitions.

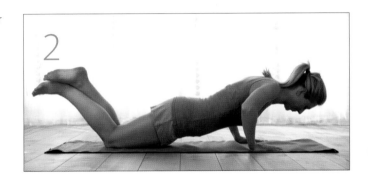

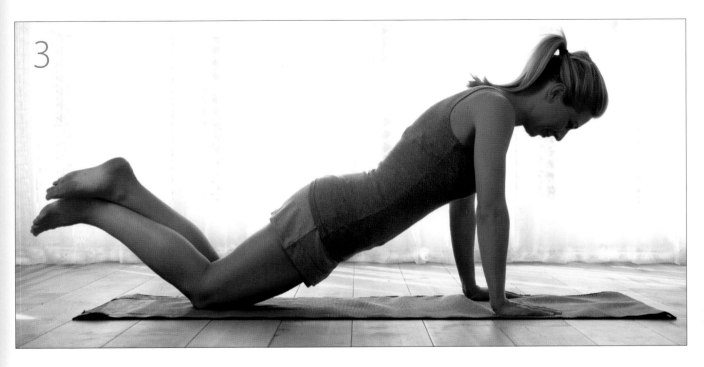

arms and shoulders

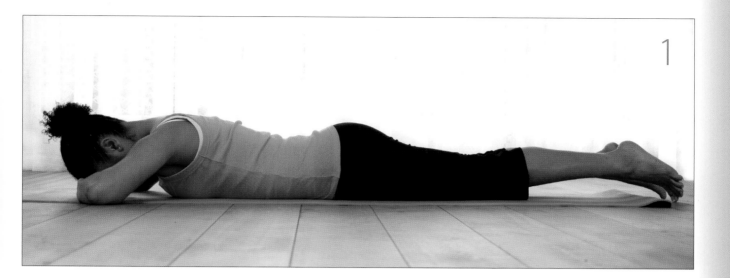

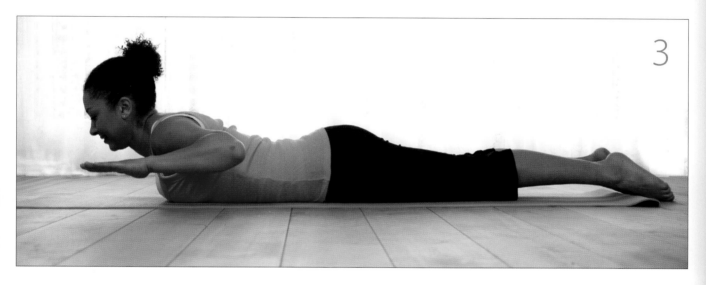

Reverse sit-up

This is a great exercise for strengthening the lower back. Adding an arm rotation to the move delivers a double toning boost to the shoulders.

1 Lie flat and face-down on the floor with your forehead resting on the backs of your hands.

2 Squeeze your buttocks and use your stomach muscles to raise your chest off the floor as far as you feel comfortable.

3 Squeeze your shoulder blades together by rotating your arms around from the shoulders so your palms are facing downward and your forearms are hovering at chest level. This will help to give the shoulders a workout, too.

4 Return your arms to the starting position and lower your chest back down to the floor. Repeat the movement. Perform ten repetitions.

WATCH POINT
Don't try to pull your chest back too far or it will force your lower back to arch and put a strain on the muscles. Just do what feels comfortable.

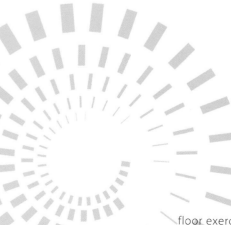

Open flyer

This floor exercise will tone through your chest, shoulders, and arms while working on your upper body strength and flexibility.

1 Lie on the mat. Hold a weight in each hand over your chest with your arms up and your palms facing each other.

2 Keeping your elbows slightly bent, lower your arms out to the sides and bring them down until they're level with your chest.

3 Keep your elbows in a fixed position and avoid lowering the weights too low.

4 Squeeze your chest to bring your arms back up, as though you're hugging a tree. Repeat the exercise ten times.

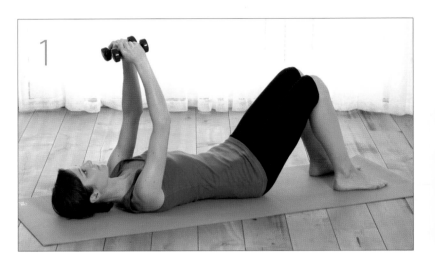

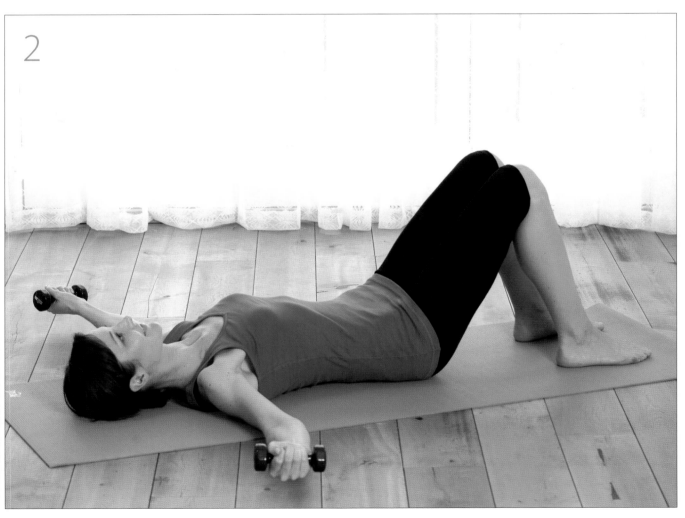

shoulders, chest, and arms

Super chest toner

This is a great exercise to work deep into the chest muscles, which can help to support and lift the bust muscles, as well as increase your range of flexibility through your shoulders.

WATCH POINT
By keeping your navel drawn down tight toward your spine, you will protect your back throughout this workout.
Doing this will also tone your deepest abdominal muscles.

1 Lie on the mat, face-up, with your knees bent and feet firmly on the floor.

2 Holding a weight in each hand, bend your arms out to the side so they rest on the floor, elbows in line with your shoulders and bent, to form an L-shape.

3 Slowly lift your arms off the floor while maintaining the bend and aim to bring both arms to meet directly in line with your face. Hold for a couple of seconds, then slowly lower back to the floor and repeat ten times.

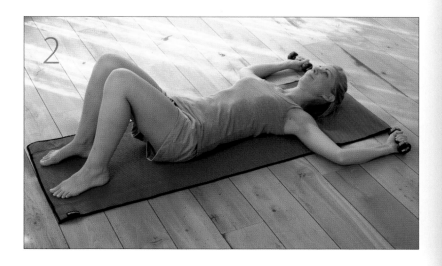

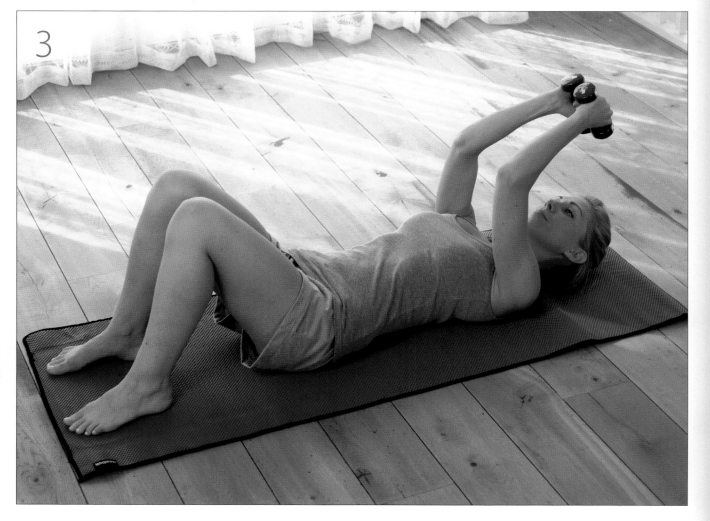

Dumbbell press

This exercise is great for toning the muscles in your chest and around your collarbone to help give you a slinky look. Make this exercise a priority if you're aiming to squeeze into a strapless dress in two weeks time!

1 Lie on your back, with your knees bent and feet flat on the floor, holding a dumbbell or tin of soup in each hand.

2 Bend your elbows and rest your hands by your armpits, so they're hovering just above your shoulders.

3 Extend your arms into the air at a right angle to your body, holding the dumbbells directly above your shoulders with your palms facing away from you.

4 Pull in your abdominals and tilt your chin toward your chest

5 Release your chin, then bend your elbows and bring your hands back to the starting position. Pause for one second, then repeat. Aim to do ten repetitions, or more if you are able.

WATCH POINT
Push from the shoulders as you extend your arms, for maximum effect. Also, make sure your lower back is pushed into the floor all the time throughout this exercise.

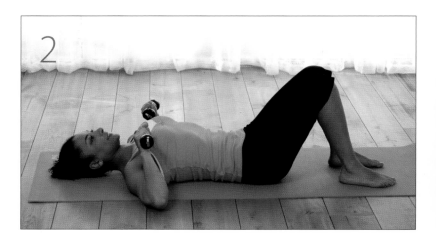

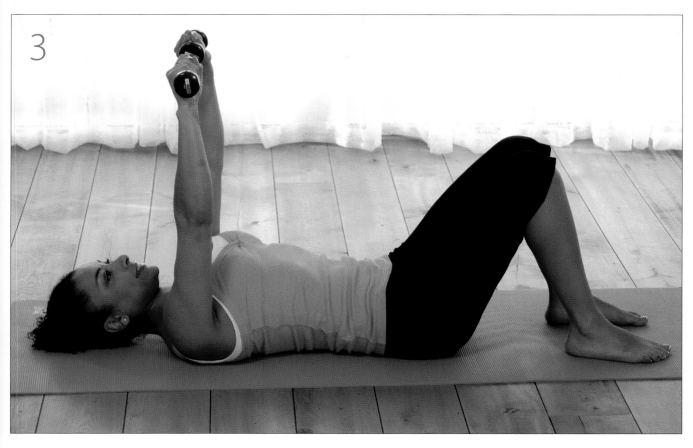

shoulders and chest

Belly tightener

Exercising in this position means you are working against gravity, making your muscles work even harder. Remember to keep your elbows soft, not locked. This is also known as abdominal hollowing and helps to shorten the abdominal muscles, which is good for your posture and creates the appearance of a flatter stomach.

1 Kneel down on all fours (the "box" position) with your hands shoulder-width apart, your elbows slightly bent, and your knees under your hips. Keep your head in line with the rest of your body and look down at the floor, making sure that your chin isn't tucked tightly into your chest.

2 Relax your abdominal muscles, then slowly draw in your navel toward your spine.

3 Hold the muscles in for a count of ten, then slowly relax. Repeat the movement ten times. Make sure you breathe slowly and steadily throughout this exercise.

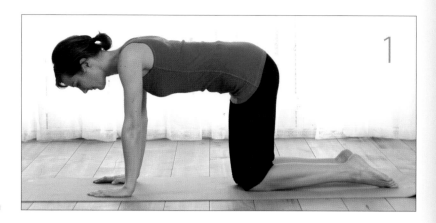

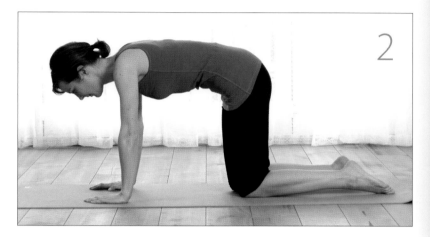

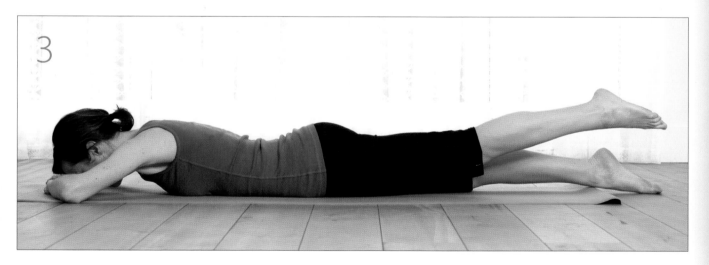

Prone leg raise

Leg raises stretch and strengthen your abs, lengthen your lower spine, and strengthen your lower back. Keep your hip bones down on the floor as you do this exercise.

1 Lie on the floor with your arms folded in front of you, your head resting on top of your arms.

2 Keep your pelvis in neutral and gently tighten your abdominal muscles so that your pubic bone is pressing down into the floor. Keep your buttock muscles tight, too.

3 Lift one leg about 6 in (15 cm) off the floor. Hold for a count of five, then release and raise the other leg. Perform ten repetitions on each leg.

Swan

This lengthens and strengthens your spine, as well as working your abs. To maintain the tension in your abdominals during this exercise, imagine that you are trying to lift your stomach off the ground.

1 Lie on your front with your arms extended in front of you and your legs extended behind.

2 Keep your spine in neutral and tighten your abdominal muscles. You should feel your pubic bone pressing down into the floor.

3 Raise your shoulders and feet a few inches off the ground and hold for a count of ten, then release. Perform five repetitions.

WATCH POINT
Consult a doctor before doing this exercise if you have ever had any lower-back problems.

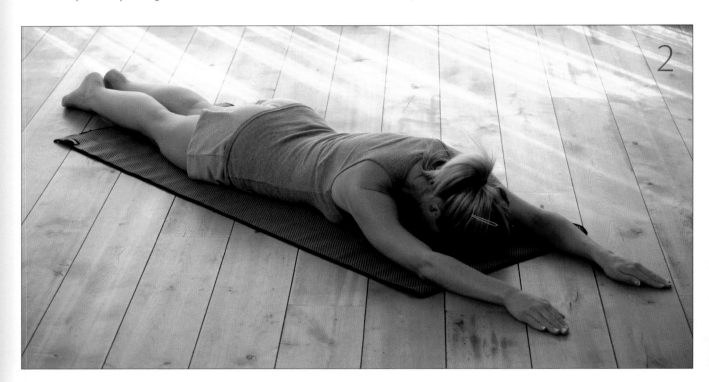

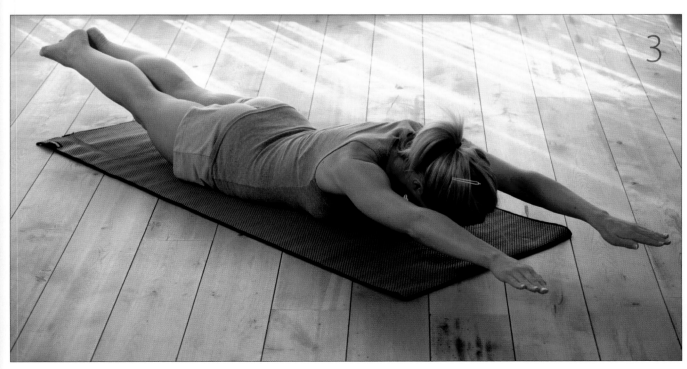

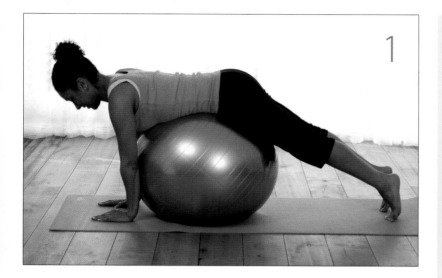

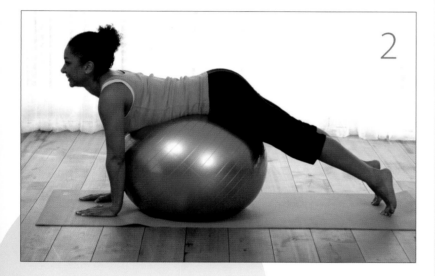

Swan—variation using an exercise ball

Performing this move on an exercise ball strengthens and stretches your back. Don't attempt this exercise if you feel any discomfort in your lower back; stop immediately.

1 Lie with the ball under your stomach and pelvis. Plant your curled toes on the floor, hip-width apart, and keep your legs straight. Place your hands on the floor, shoulder-width apart.

2 Tighten your abdominal muscles and lift your head so that there is a long line from your head to your heels. Slowly push your pelvis into the ball as you look up and extend your spine away from the ball.

3 Hold this extended position for a count of five, then release. Perform at least three repetitions.

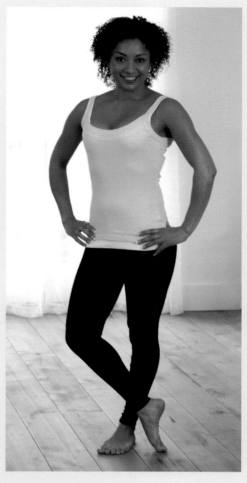

WORKING WITH YOUR BODY SHAPE

We all have a unique bone structure and body shape that, frankly, we cannot change. Some of us are genetically programed to be very slender (ectomorphs), others are curvaceous with a tendency to gain weight (endomorphs), while others tend to be athletic and trim (mesomorphs).

Consider your body shape before embarking on your fitness routine—if you are a natural endomorph, no amount of exercise or dieting will give you a waif-like, ectomorphic look.

Furthermore, women are naturally designed to store fat on the hips and thighs to protect the reproductive organs—that is, until the menopause, after which they will store fat around the midsection, just like men!

back and stomach

Easy plank (tension hold)

Holding your body in a three-quarters plank shape strengthens the deep transverse muscles that cross the stomach area. Keeping your knees on the floor makes this exercise much easier than the traditional plank, to which you can progress when you feel ready.

1 Adopt a traditional press-up position but keep your knees on the floor and your feet in the air. Your fingers should point forward, your elbows stay straight but not locked, your head should be in line with your body, and your feet together. Keep your shoulder blades drawn into your back and make sure you don't dip in the middle or raise your bottom in the air.

2 Hold this position for a count of ten, breathing regularly throughout. Repeat ten times.

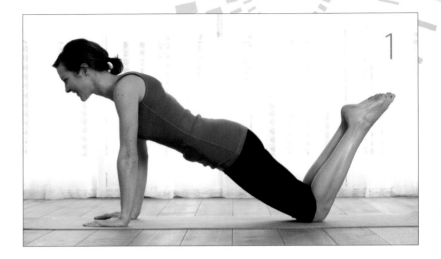

Simple pelvic tilt

This exercise tightens the abdominal muscles without putting any strain on your back. It's a simple way to tone and strengthen your abdominal area.

1 Lie on your back with your knees bent and feet flat on the floor, hip-width apart, and your spine in neutral position. Rest your arms by your sides, palms facing the floor, and gradually tighten your abdominal muscles.

2 Press your lower back down into the floor and gently tilt your pelvis so that the pubic bone rises, then tilt it back down.

3 Repeat the movement ten times, using a slow, steady rhythm.

WATCH POINT
This easy exercise is particularly good if you're trying to shape up post-pregnancy.

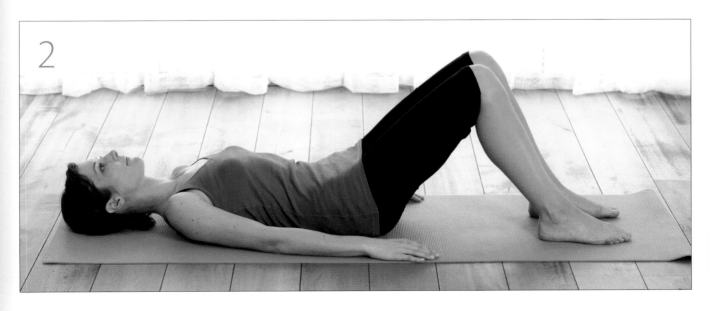

stomach

Plank

This exercise doesn't sound or look too taxing but, if you do it right, you'll find that it's one of the most intense exercises in this book, and very effective at toning the abdominal muscles. Many people, especially beginners, find this difficult to hold for long periods of time, so see how you get on. Initially, aim to hold the position for ten seconds, but if you exercise regularly, once you become fitter, you should be able to hold the position for a full 30 seconds.

1 Lie on the floor on your front, resting your forehead on the backs of your hands.

2 Keeping your elbows bent, slide your hands across the floor, rotating from the shoulders, until you find your perfect "press-up" position with your hands placed either side of your chest.

3 Curl your toes underneath you and push up off the floor with your hands. Keep your elbows soft to stop them locking, and keep your neck and head relaxed and in line with your spine.

4 Hold the pose for ten seconds, then gently lower yourself back down to the floor again. Remember to breathe during the exercise. Start by doing three sets of ten seconds. As you become fitter, gradually try to increase the time that you hold the Plank to a full 30 seconds.

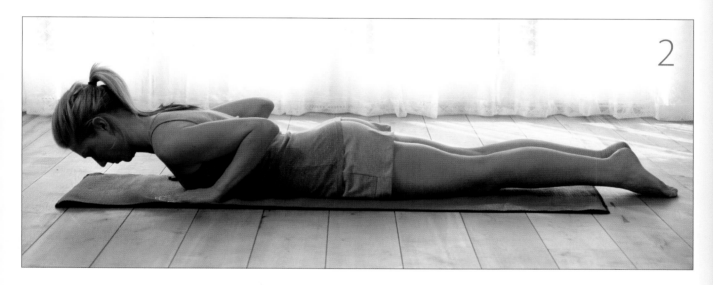

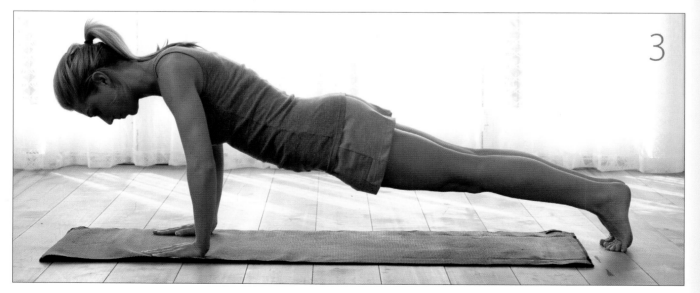

stomach

Abdominal curl

Say farewell to sloppy sit-ups—a few properly executed curl-ups will work wonders in helping you achieve a flatter stomach. This exercise will tone the rectus abdominis muscle, which runs down the front of your stomach. As you lift your head and shoulders, this muscle contracts at both ends. Avoid this type of exercise, however, if you have neck problems.

1 Lie on your back with a firm, flat pillow or a small towel underneath your head. Keep your feet hip-width apart, parallel and firmly on the floor, and your knees bent. Rest your hands on your thighs.

2 Set your spine in the neutral position and tighten your abdominal muscles. Flex your spine to lift your head and shoulders gently about 30 degrees off the floor. Your hands will slide up toward your knees as you curl. Keep your lower back in contact with the floor at all times.

3 Slowly curl back down in a continuous movement. To make this exercise more challenging, put your hands across your chest as you curl. When this becomes easy, you can place your hands at the sides of your head to increase the resistance against which you are working. Repeat the exercise ten times.

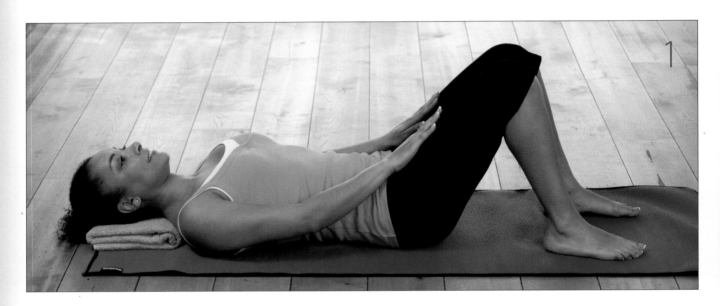

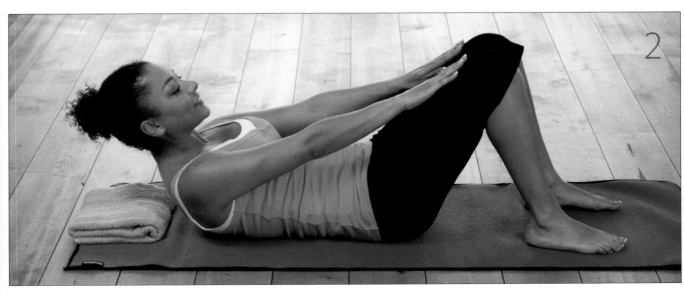

stomach

Crunches

This is an intense workout for your stomach muscles and a great way of getting a washboard-flat abdomen.

1 Lie on the floor, knees bent and feet (apart) flat on the floor in line with your hips. Make sure that your lower back is pressed into the floor. Put your hands behind your head to support your neck.

2 Engage your stomach muscles, by pulling your abdominals toward your spine, and lift your upper body off the floor as far as you can without arching your lower back. You may find that you can't get up very high, but it's the effort of moving that counts, so make sure that you're pushing yourself as hard as you comfortably can. With practice, you may be able to sit up completely.

3 When you can't go any farther, pause for one second. Then gently lower yourself back down into the starting position and repeat five times. Try to do as many sets of five as possible, with a brief rest between.

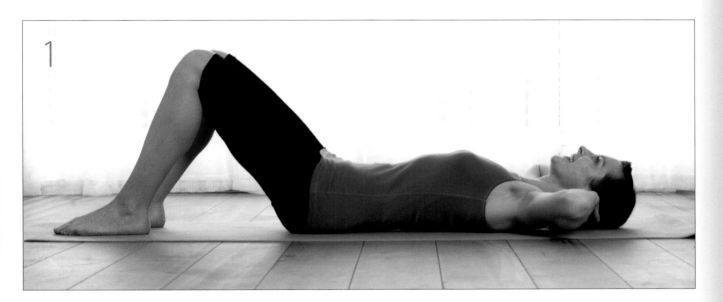

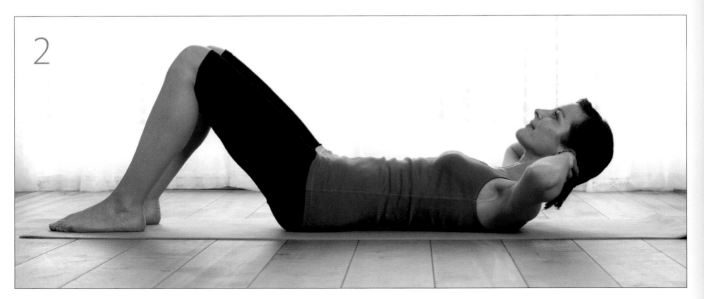

stomach

Bicycle

This is similar to the Crunches exercise, but crossing your elbow to the opposite knee targets the oblique muscles instead, which are found at the side of the waist. Practicing this exercise will help to give you a smaller, more defined middle. This exercise is great for your waist but you may find it too hard if you're a beginner. However, you should be able to do it after a few weeks of stomach-toning exercise.

1 Lie on the floor with your knees bent and feet resting flat on the floor.

2 Rest your hands behind your head, lift your right foot off the floor and bring your right knee toward your chest.

3 Using your stomach muscles, lift your upper body off the floor, making sure that your lower back stays firmly on the floor.

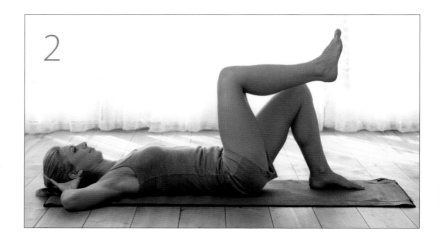

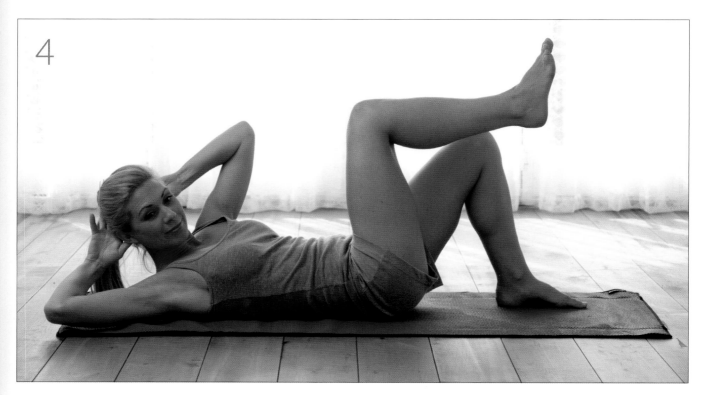

4 Reach forward and rotate from the waist slightly in order to bring your left elbow toward your right knee. They don't have to touch.

5 Pause for one second then return to the starting position. Repeat the movement, bringing your right knee toward your left elbow. Continue the exercise on alternate sides for 30 seconds. Aim to do as many repetitions as you can in 30 seconds—around 10 or 12. Take a short rest if you have to—for example, pause briefly between sets of five.

stomach

Lower abdominal raise

This is a challenging exercise that will really work your deep abdominal muscles. If it seems easy, then you're not doing it properly!

1 Lie on your back with your knees bent, feet flat on the floor and hip-width apart. Make sure your spine is in neutral. Keep your arms by your sides with the palms facing upward.

2 Lift your legs into the air at an angle of 90 degrees to your body.

3 Tighten your abdominal muscles and slowly lower one foot to the floor then bring it back up again. Repeat this exercise using the other leg. Aim to build up to ten repetitions on each side.

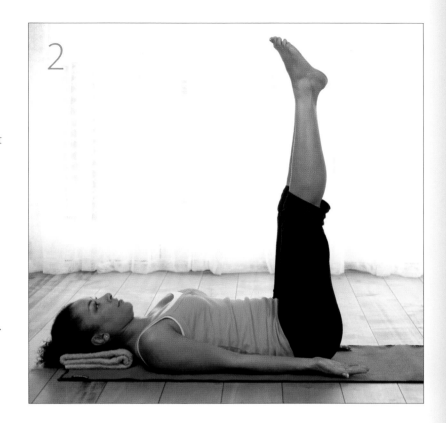

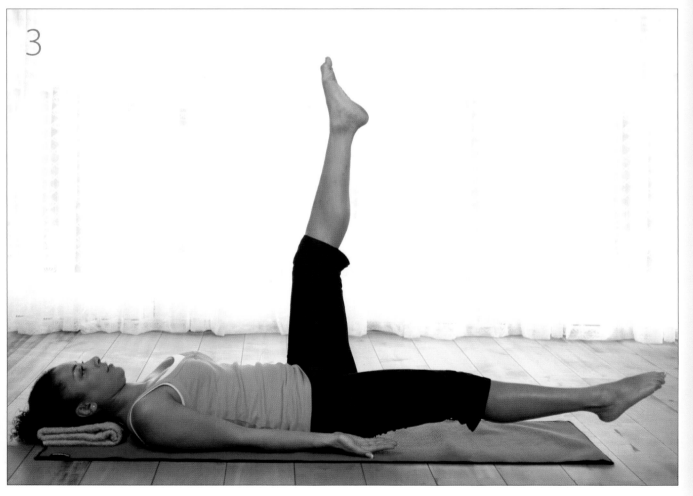

stomach

Basic abdominal exercise using a ball

This exercise using an exercise ball will prepare you for more difficult abdominal workouts. It works the muscles that support and strengthen your lower spine which play an important part in keeping your pelvis stable and spine aligned. Try to keep your pelvis in neutral.

1 Lie on the floor with your feet on the ball, with your knees bent and legs together.

2 Place your hands on your hip bones to stabilize your pelvis.

3 Very gently, breathe in and let your knees fall open to hip-width apart.

4 As you breathe out, bring your legs back together, pulling your stomach in so that your navel is being drawn down and into your spine. Repeat ten times.

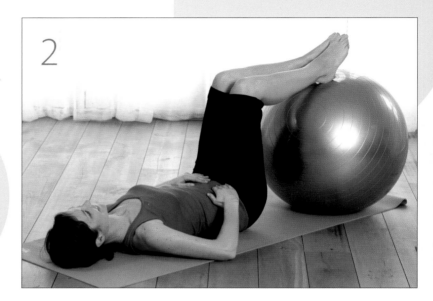

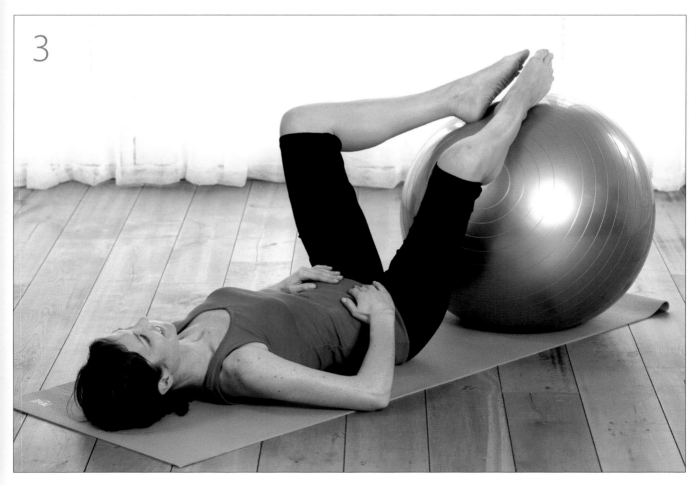

Leg lift

Exercising on all fours makes your muscles work harder because they're working against gravity. Keep all movements smooth and controlled for best results and don't let your back sag or arch. This lateral thigh raise works the outer thigh muscles (hip abductors).

1 To start, kneel in the "box" position (on all fours) and keep your back straight. Tighten your abdominal muscles to support your back.

2 Lift your left leg out to the side—you will feel the muscles at the side of the thigh and hip working to lift your leg. Hold for a count of two.

3 Slowly lower your leg to the start position. Do ten repetitions on one leg, then repeat using the other leg.

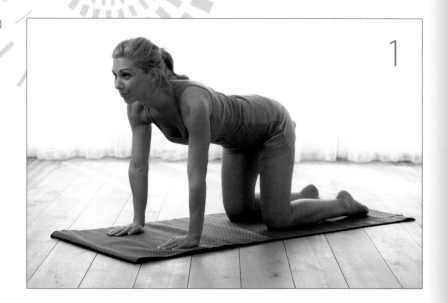

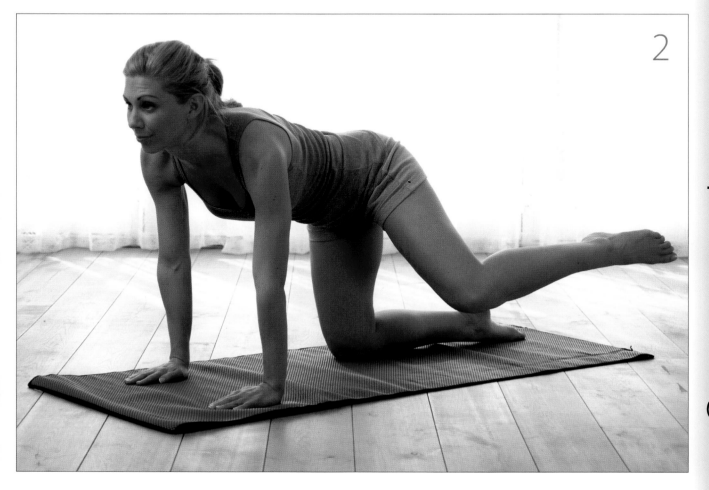

One-hip leg extension

This exercise works the hip extensors (gluteals). To increase the intensity, straighten out the leg you are working, but remember to keep the knee soft.

1 Get into the box position on all fours and keep your back straight.

2 Tighten your abdominal muscles to protect your back. Tense your buttocks.

3 Lift your right leg upward with your knee bent and your thigh parallel to the floor.

4 Gently lift your thigh about 2 in (5 cm) up and then lower again. Lower the leg back to the floor, then do all your repetitions on one leg. Repeat the exercise with the other leg.

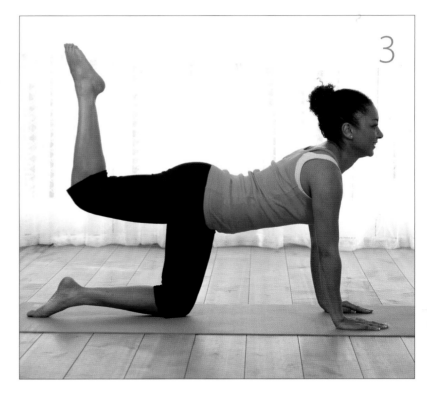

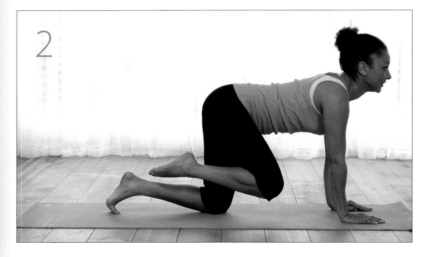

Kneeling kick-back

This exercise works your quadriceps.

1 Get down on all fours and pull in your stomach muscles to protect your back.

2 Raise your right leg off the floor, and with your knee bent, bring it into your body, then stretch it out backward so that it is in line with your body with the foot flexed.

3 Pull the leg back in and take it back out again. Perform ten repetitions on one leg, then repeat using the other leg.

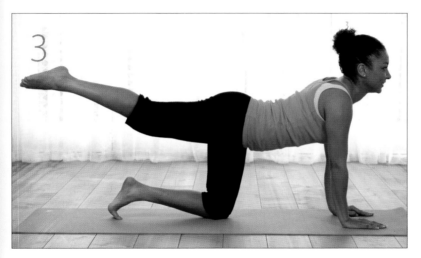

WATCH POINT
Don't kick back vigorously because this builds up momentum, which can place stress on your lower back muscles.

Scissors

This exercise is fabulous for toning your inner thighs and tightening up your stomach muscles.

1 Lie on your back with your legs straight up in the air. Keep your spine in neutral and tighten your abdominal muscles to protect your back.

2 Make a "V" shape with your legs and then, in a smooth, continuous motion, cross your left leg in front of your right leg, then switch sides in a scissor-like motion. Continue for 30 seconds.

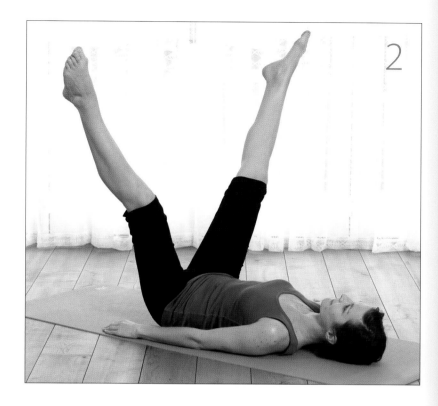

2

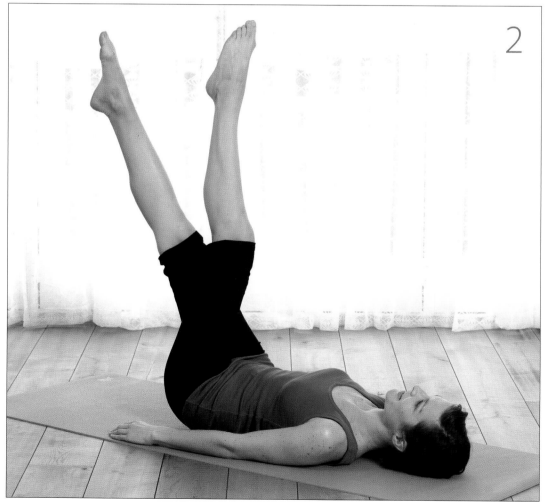

2

WATCH POINT
Make sure your spine is in the right position when you are exercising. If you exercise with your pelvis and spine misplaced— either pressed too far into the floor or arched—you may put stress on your lower back and create muscle imbalance.

stomach and thighs

Outer thigh lift

These side-lying exercises work the abductor muscles at the side of the thighs. Make sure you perform each move slowly and in a controlled way to really work the muscles to the full.

1 Lie on your right side with your body in a straight line and your thighs and feet together. Prop yourself up with your right arm and rest your left hand on the floor in front of you. Tighten your stomach muscles by drawing your navel in toward your spine—this will help to protect your back.

2 Bend both knees. Lift up the top leg, then lower, squeezing your buttocks together as you raise and lower your leg.

3 Do ten repetitions on one side, then repeat on the other side of your body.

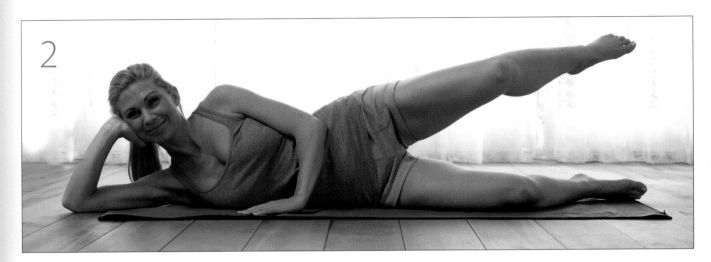

Straight-legged outer thigh lift

Keep your back straight, your hips facing forward, and breathe regularly throughout.

1 Lie on your side with your lower leg bent and your top leg straight but with the knee soft rather than locked. Your body should be in a straight line and your thighs and knees together. Prop yourself up on your elbow with your head resting on your hand and place the other hand in front of you for support. Keep your stomach muscles pulled in to protect your back.

2 Raise your top leg, then lower, squeezing your buttock muscles as you do so. If you are in the correct position, you shouldn't be able to lift your leg more than 45 degrees.

3 Do ten repetitions on one side, then repeat them on the other side of your body.

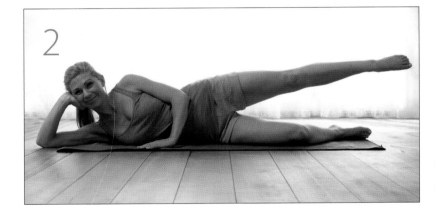

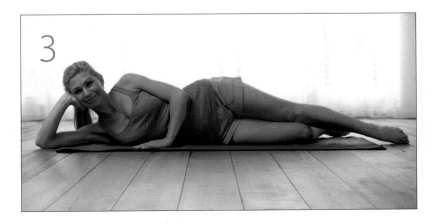

thighs and hips

Inner thigh lift

Remember to keep your spine in neutral and your stomach muscles tightened throughout. You don't have to tense your buttocks as you do this but it's good to work your gluteals whenever you can.

1 Lie on one side with your hips facing forward and your body in a straight line. Prop yourself up on your elbow with your head resting on your hand and place the other hand on the floor in front of you for support.

2 Tighten your stomach muscles by gently drawing in your navel toward your spine to protect your back.

3 Bend your top leg so that the knee touches the floor in front of you.

4 Raise the bottom extended leg, keeping the knee soft (slightly bent), then lower it.

5 Do ten repetitions on one side, then repeat them on the other side of your body.

WATCH POINT
This exercise may look easy, but it will really work to tighten and strengthen the hips and thighs.

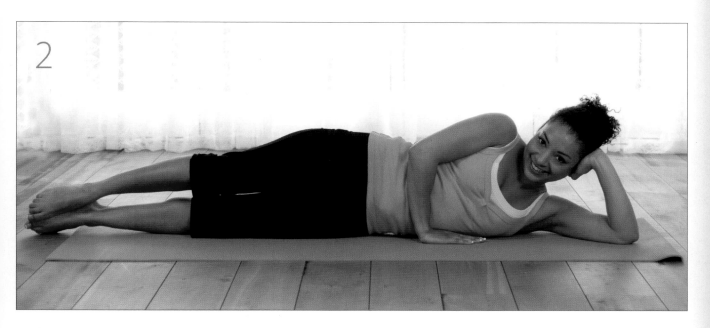

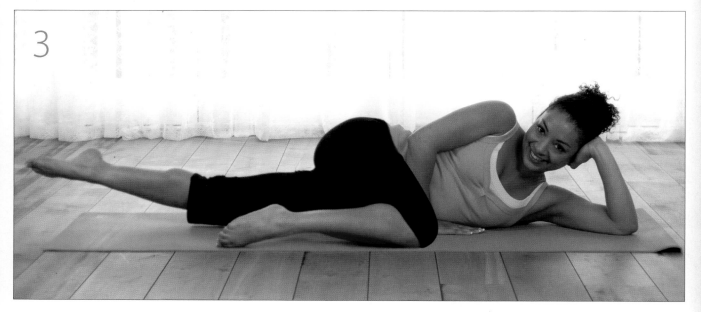

thighs and hips

Basic bridge

Bridges and planks are static exercises that enable you to assess your core strength by the length of time you are able to hold the positions. However, they are only effective if you maintain a flat line from your shoulders to your feet. You need to perfect this exercise in order to improve the stability of the trunk muscles before you can move on to more challenging movements.

1 Lie on your back with your knees bent, feet parallel, hip-width apart. Keep your arms close by your sides with palms on the mat.

2 Tighten your abdominal muscles and tilt your pelvis slowly upward as you would do in a pelvic tilt (see page 70).

3 Press your feet down firmly and gently lift your hips, lower-, and mid-back off the floor. Aim to align your hips with your thighs and body.

4 Hold for a count of ten, then release and lower slowly to the floor. Relax. Perform two repetitions. As you become fitter, you will be able to hold the position for longer.

WATCH POINT
Use your hands for balance but don't push yourself up.

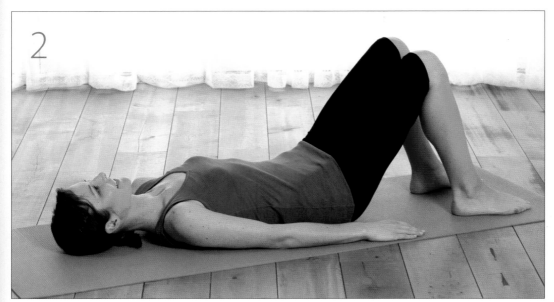

2

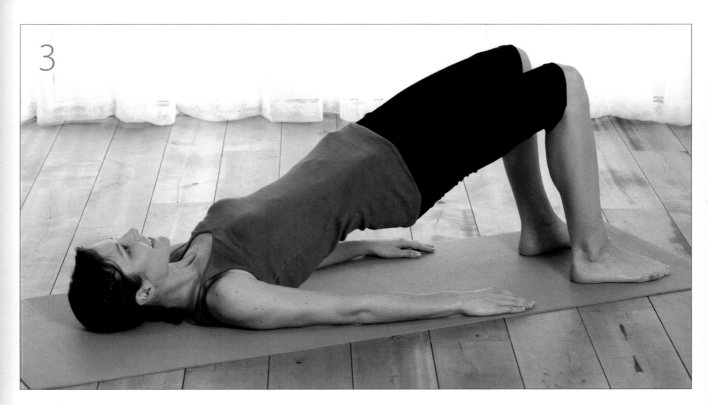

3

Basic bridge—variation using an exercise ball

Bridging using an exercise ball makes your rectus abdominis and external obliques work harder.

1 Lie on your back with your arms by your sides. Place your legs on the ball so that it is resting under your calf muscles.

2 Tighten your abdominal muscles and lift your hips off the floor until your body is diagonal from shoulders to knees.

3 Hold for a count of ten, then release and lower slowly to the floor. Relax, then perform two repetitions. As you become fitter, you will be able to hold the position for longer.

WATCH POINT
Take care not to overarch your back or let it sag, and remember to keep your breathing steady and controlled.

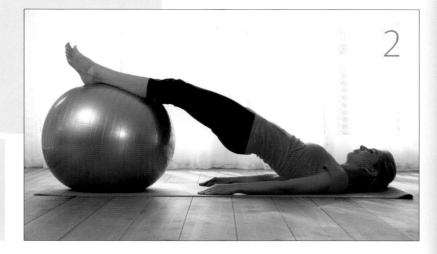

Bridge squeeze

Although the bridge squeeze looks similar to the basic bridge, this buttock-clenching exercise is designed to make the buttock muscles work to support your back. If you feel a strong contraction in your hamstrings or any strain in your lower back, then you are not using your buttock muscles properly.

1 Lie on your back with your knees bent and feet slightly apart. Tighten your abdominal muscles by gently drawing in your navel toward your spine. This will protect your back muscles.

2 Curl your bottom off the floor, lifting your pelvis until your knees, hips, and chest are in line.

3 Hold this for a count of ten, squeezing your buttock muscles to support the bridge position. Release and repeat once more. As you become fitter, you will be able to hold the position for longer.

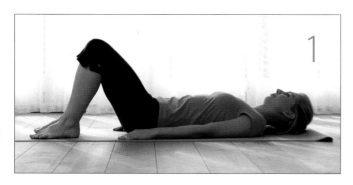

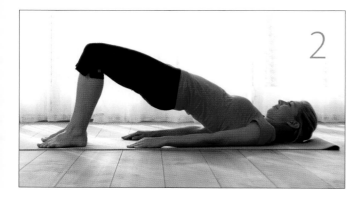

stomach and buttocks

Rear leg raise

This exercise will help to strengthen and tone both the gluteus maximus (the major muscles in the buttocks, which are also known as the glutes) and also the lower back.

1 Lie on the floor with your forehead resting on the backs of your hands. Make sure your spine is in line with your neck.

2 Squeeze your buttocks—it will make the exercise harder and more effective. Then, engage your abdominal muscles and gently lift your left leg off the floor until you feel the muscles working in your buttocks. Keep your leg straight and your knee soft. You shouldn't feel any pain in your lower back.

3 Lower your left leg back into the starting position, then repeat the movement with your right leg and again with your left and so on. Aim to complete around three sets of ten. You can do five sets of six with a slight pause between if you prefer.

KEEPING UP YOUR MOTIVATION

All too often people start a new exercise regime burning with enthusiasm, only for it to peter out very quickly to the point where they can't be bothered to do anything at all. When you start your toning program, be realistic about how and when you can do it.

You need to set aside a regular slot for your exercise routine so that it becomes a natural and automatic part of your everyday routine. But if you do miss several days, don't become disheartened and give up—a little exercise even on a very irregular basis is still better than nothing at all.

WATCH POINT
Don't try to lift your leg too high or it will force your back to arch and put a strain on the muscles.

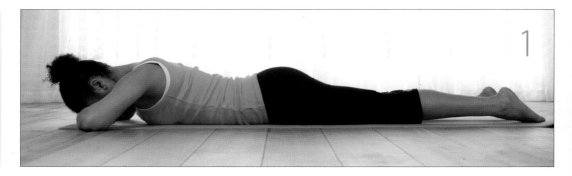

1

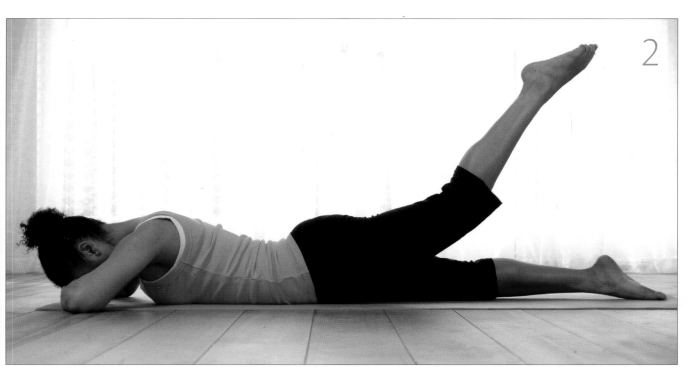

2

buttocks and lower back

Basic buttock toner using an exercise ball

Buttock muscles are not just for sitting on—they also help to move your legs. Tension in the gluteals can lead to back problems and poor posture, so it's very important to keep these muscles flexible and strong.

1 Lie on the ball with your arms shoulder-width apart with the palms of your hands planted on the floor. Keep your head and neck aligned with your spine. Your toes should be touching the floor with your feet flexed for balance.

2 Slowly lift your left leg until it is pointing out straight behind you, keeping the buttock muscles clenched as you do so. Hold for a count of five. Return to the starting position and repeat on the other side. Aim to perform five repetitions on each side.

3 When you are used to this exercise and feel able to perform a more challenging movement, slowly lift both legs until they are pointing out straight behind you, keeping the buttock muscles clenched as you do so. Hold for a count of five. Return to the starting position.

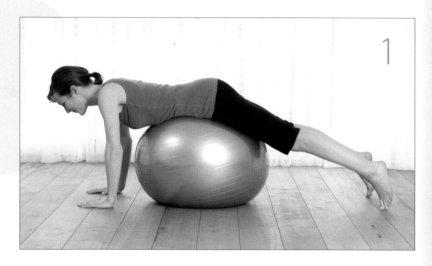

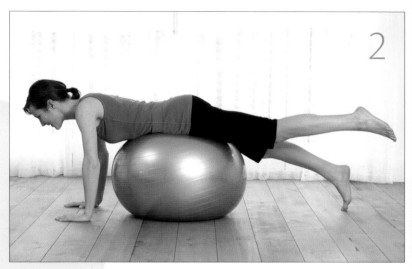

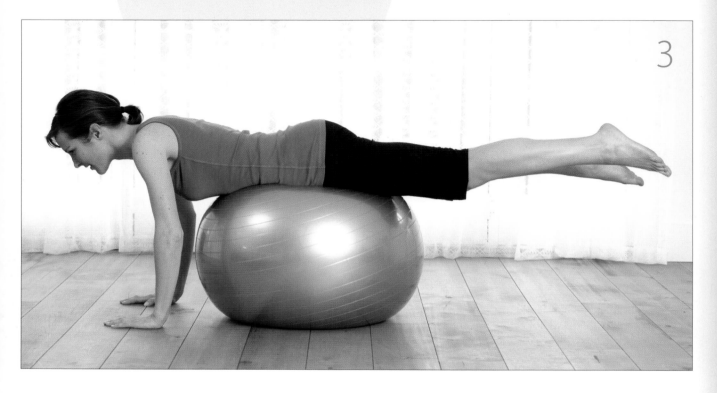

buttocks

COOL DOWN AND STRETCH

Just as important as warming up before exercising is cooling down afterward. Help your body return to normal in a gentle way by taking the time to perform cooling-down stretches at the end of an exercise session. As well as helping to prevent dizziness and a sudden drop in body temperature (which can make you feel unwell), cooling down realigns working muscles to their normal position to prevent post-exercise tightness and stiffness. Hold each stretch for as long as is comfortable for you and repeat each exercise a few times until you can feel the full benefit of the stretch.

Standing waist stretch

1 Stand with your legs fairly wide apart, knees soft. Turn your left foot outward. Keep your right leg straight with the foot flat on the floor and pointing forward. Rest your left palm lighty on your left thigh.

2 Lift your right arm above your head and lean toward your left side, sliding your left hand slowly down your leg. Keep your back straight and do not overstretch. Hold for a count of ten. Repeat on the other side.

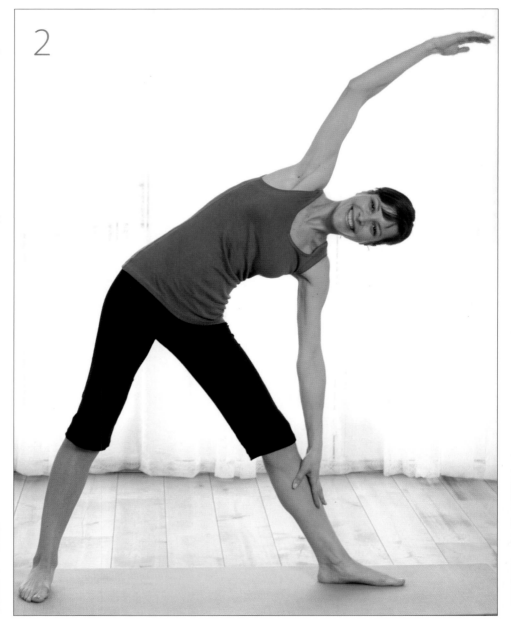

2

WATCH POINT
Don't lean too far over—you should feel a stretch but it shouldn't hurt.

cool down

Sitting body twister

1 Sit on the floor with your legs straight out in front of you. Bend your right leg and cross it over your left knee.

2 Gently rotate your trunk and head toward your left as far as is comfortable, keeping your buttocks on the floor throughout.

3 Hold for a count of ten, then release and return to the starting position. Repeat on the other side.

WATCH POINT
Stretch only as far as is comfortable.

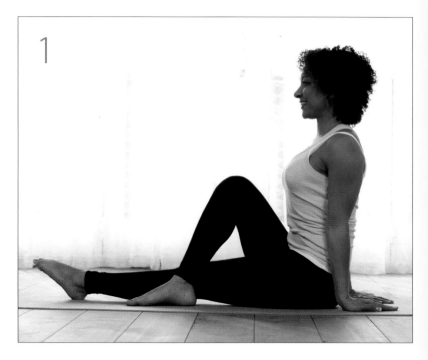

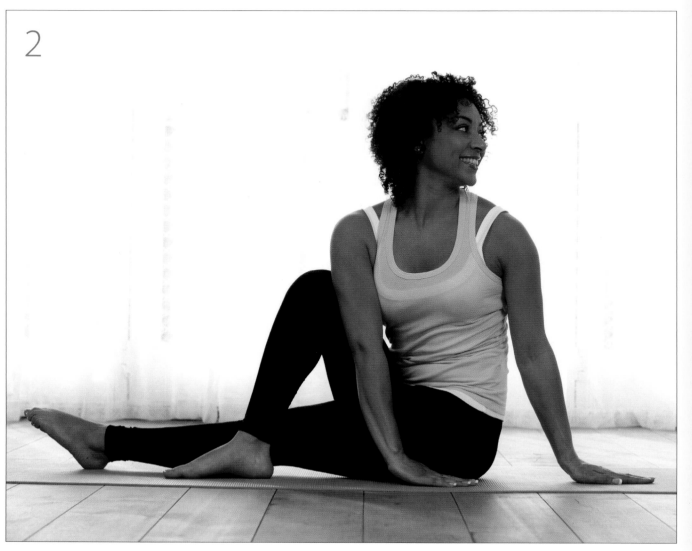

Leg lift and cross

1 Lie on your back with your legs out straight and your arms stretched out to the sides.

2 Breathe in to prepare, and tighten your abdominal muscles. Lift your right leg up to the ceiling as you breathe out, and flex your foot.

3 Using your abdominal muscles to control and pace the movement, lower your leg slowly across your body over to the left side until the foot gently touches the floor.

4 Hold for a count of 20, then slowly return to the starting position. Repeat on the other side.

WATCH POINT
If you can't take your foot all the way to the floor, bend your arm up to meet your foot and rest the foot on your hand.

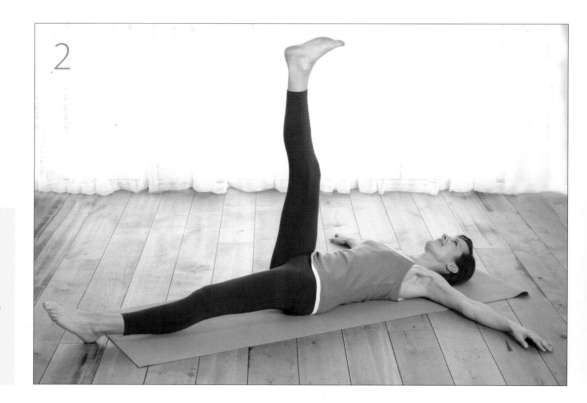

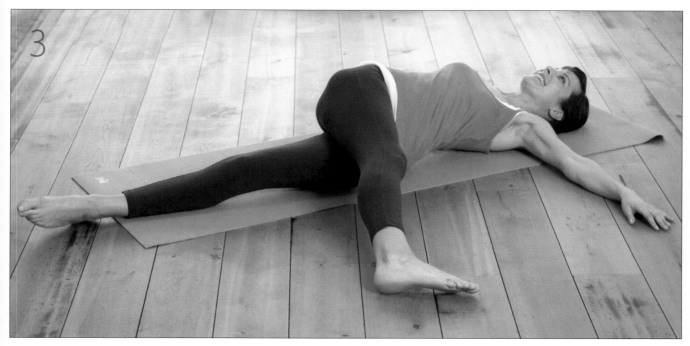

Hip and thigh stretch

1 Kneel with one knee above the ankle and foot flat on the floor, and stretch your other leg behind you so that the knee gently touches the floor.

2 Place your hands on your front knee to balance yourself. Hold this position for a count of ten, then repeat with the other leg.

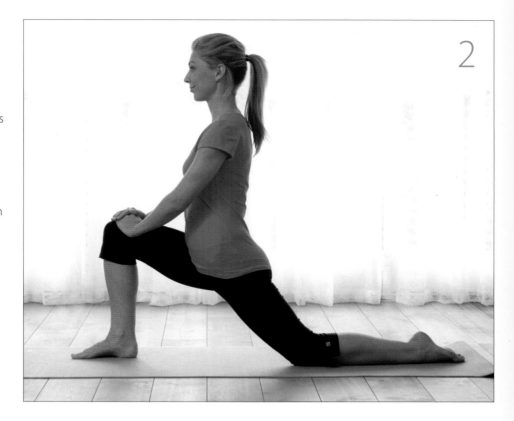

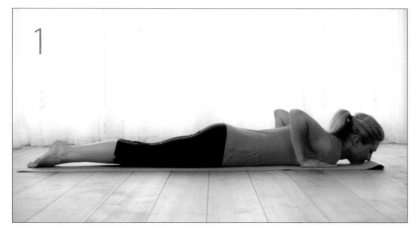

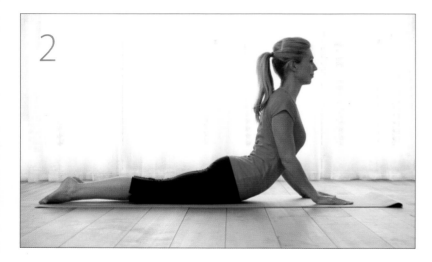

Cobra stretch

This modified yoga position is excellent for stretching your stomach muscles.

1 Lie on your front on the floor and put your hands underneath your shoulders.

2 Breathe in to prepare, then gently push your arms up until they are straight but your elbows are not locked. This will lift your head and chest upward and you will feel a stretch in your abdominal muscles. Your hips should stay in contact with the floor throughout.

3 Hold for a count of ten, then slowly lower yourself back to the ground.

WATCH POINT
Ensure all your movements are slow and controlled during stretching to avoid straining any muscles.

cool down

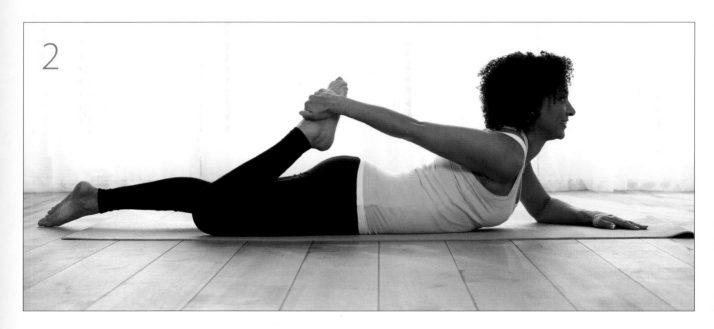

2

Lying quad stretch

1 Lie prone (face down) on the floor. Bend one knee and take hold of the foot of that leg with your hand and gently pull the foot toward your buttock.

2 Press your hip down toward the floor (which will ensure you stretch fully the rectus femoris—the quadriceps muscle that crosses the hip joint).

3 Hold the stretch for a count of ten, then release and repeat with the other leg. Don't tug on your leg; you want a gentle stretch.

Lying hamstring stretch

1 Lie on your back with your knees bent and your feet resting flat on the floor.

2 Lift one leg and grasp the back of the thigh with your hands.

3 Gently pull that leg toward your chest as far as is comfortable. Repeat with the other leg.

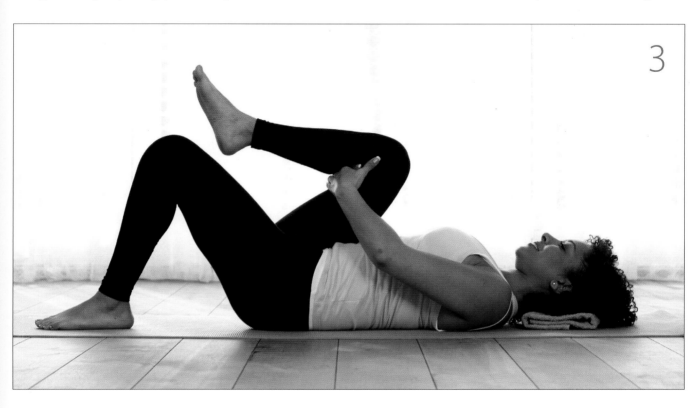

3

cool down

Knee hug

This will stretch and release the muscles in your lower back.

1 Lie on your back with your legs in the air and your knees bent. Tighten your abdominal muscles to protect your lower back.

2 Lift your knees to your chest and hold on to your shins.

3 Pull your knees in as tightly as is comfortable and hold for at least 15 seconds. Slowly release, return to the start position, and repeat a few times.

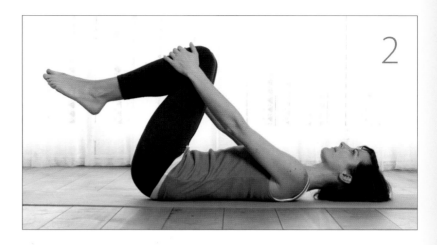

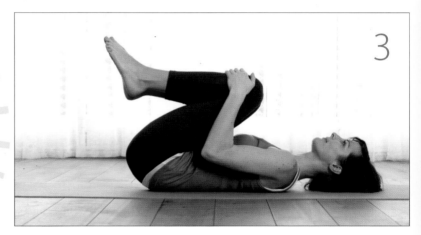

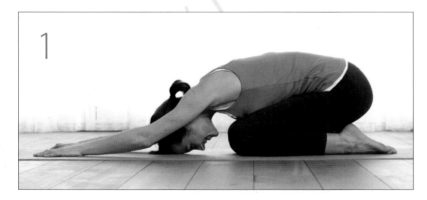

Child's pose

This classic yoga position is great for relaxing your entire back.

1 Get on all fours with your hands under your shoulders and your knees under your hips. Rock your buttocks back toward your heels, pulling your navel in against your spine as you do so. Rest your stomach on your thighs and your head on the floor.

2 Take your arms back so that your hands are close to your feet. Hold the pose for a count of 15, then relax. Repeat a few times, then slowly sit up before getting to your feet.

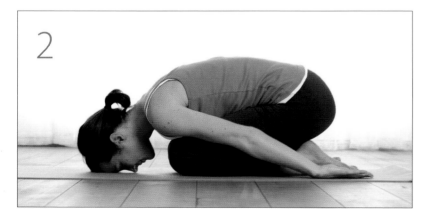

WORKOUT SUGGESTIONS

Here are some workout suggestions to get you started on your new Stay Fit, Stay Young exercise routine. Remember that it is very important to warm up properly before you begin, and if you are new to exercising, begin by doing just a few repetitions of each exercise. As your body becomes fitter, aim to perform ten repetitions of each exercise. We have created workout plans to target all the main muscle groups in the body, but you can also make up your own routines.

Full body workout 1

WARM UP AND STRETCH
Marching *page 24*
Cat stretch *page 25*
Triceps stretch *page 27*
Deltoid stretch *page 27*
Easy chest stretch *page 29*
Neck stretches *page 30*

STANDING EXERCISES
Standing wall press-up *page 33*
Chest press *page 39*
Arm opener *page 43*
Triceps extension *page 44*
Wide squat *page 46*

SEATED EXERCISES
Seated reverse abdominal curl *page 55*
Seated knee lift *page 56*

FLOOR EXERCISES
Belly tightener *page 67*
Swan *page 68*
Bicycle *page 74*
Leg lift *page 77*
Bridge squeeze *page 83*

COOL DOWN AND STRETCH
Standing waist stretch *page 86*
Leg lift and cross *page 88*
Hip and thigh stretch *page 89*
Knee hug *page 91*
Child's pose *page 91*

Full body workout 2

WARM UP AND STRETCH
Marching *page 24*
Forward bend *page 24*
Shoulder rolls *page 26*
Waist twist *page 28*
Hip circles *page 28*
Side bends *page 30*

STANDING EXERCISES
Shoulder press *page 32*
Side shoulder raise *page 34*
Arm circles *page 41*
Triceps extension *page 44*
Basic squat *page 46*
Front leg raise *page 48*
Rear leg raise *page 49*

FLOOR EXERCISES
Open flyer *page 64*
Plank *page 71*
Lower abdominal raise *page 75*
Scissors *page 79*

COOL DOWN AND STRETCH
Sitting body twister *page 87*
Cobra stretch *page 89*
Lying quad stretch *page 90*
Lying hamstring stretch *page 90*
Child's pose *page 91*

Upper body workout 1

WARM UP AND STRETCH
Marching *page 24*
Forward bend *page 24*
Shoulder rolls *page 26*
Arm swing *page 26*
Waist twist *page 28*
Side bends *page 30*

STANDING EXERCISES
Turning press *page 35*
Front raises *page 35*
Upright pull *page 38*
Bust lift *page 38*
Bicep curl *page 40*
Triceps extension *page 44*
Triceps kick-back *page 45*

SEATED EXERCISES
Bent-over arm shaper *page 53*

FLOOR EXERCISES
Press-ups *page 62*
Super chest toner *page 65*
Dumbbell press *page 66*

COOL DOWN AND STRETCH
Standing waist stretch *page 86*
Sitting body twister *page 87*
Cobra stretch *page 89*
Knee hug *page 91*
Child's pose *page 91*

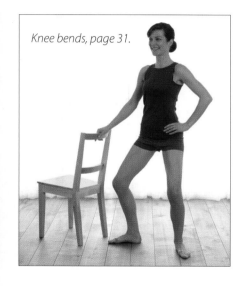

Knee bends, page 31.

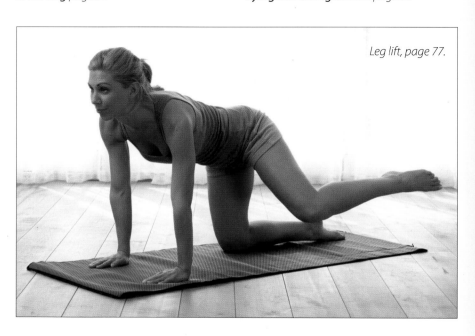

Leg lift, page 77.

workout

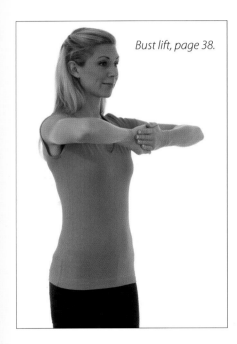

Bust lift, page 38.

Workout using floor exercises

WARM UP AND STRETCH

FLOOR EXERCISES

COOL DOWN AND STRETCH

Workout using standing exercises

WARM UP AND STRETCH

STANDING EXERCISES

COOL DOWN AND STRETCH

Abdominal workout

WARM UP AND STRETCH

FLOOR EXERCISES

COOL DOWN AND STRETCH

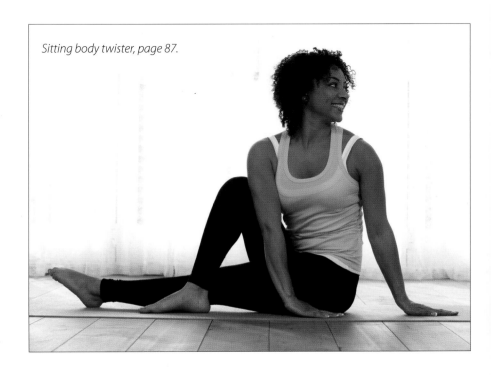

Sitting body twister, page 87.

workout

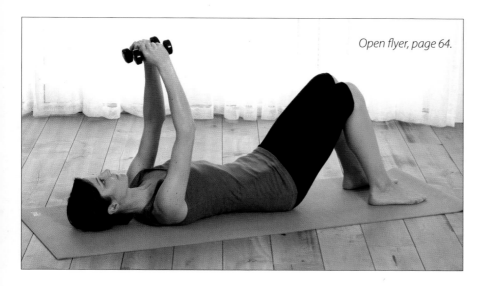

Open flyer, page 64.

Workout using an exercise ball

WARM UP AND STRETCH
Marching *page 24*
Forward bend *page 24*
Waist twist *page 28*
Easy chest stretch *page 29*
Neck stretches *page 30*
Side bends *page 30*

STANDING EXERCISES
Reach and squat *page 36*
Double shoulder stretch *page 37*
Squat variation *page 47*

SEATED EXERCISES
Sitting balance *page 60*
Toe taps *page 60*
Hip circles *page 61*

FLOOR EXERCISES
Swan variation *page 69*
Basic abdominal exercise *page 76*
Basic bridge variation *page 83*
Basic buttock toner *page 85*

COOL DOWN AND STRETCH
Standing waist stretch *page 86*
Sitting body twister *page 87*
Leg lift and cross *page 88*
Hip and thigh stretch *page 89*
Cobra stretch *page 89*

Workout using weights

WARM UP AND STRETCH
Marching *page 24*
Shoulder rolls *page 26*
Arm swing *page 26*
Triceps stretch *page 27*
Deltoid stretch *page 27*
Easy chest stretch *page 29*

STANDING EXERCISES
Shoulder press *page 32*
Side shoulder raise *page 34*
Turning press *page 35*
Front raises *page 35*
Upright pull *page 38*
Bicep curl *page 40*
Triceps extension *page 44*

SEATED EXERCISES
Bent-over arm shaper *page 53*

FLOOR EXERCISES
Open flyer *page 64*
Super chest toner *page 65*
Dumbbell press *page 66*

COOL DOWN AND STRETCH
Standing waist stretch *page 86*
Sitting body twister *page 87*
Cobra stretch *page 89*
Knee hug *page 91*
Child's pose *page 91*

Workout using a chair

WARM UP AND STRETCH
Marching *page 24*
Hip circles *page 28*
Easy chest stretch *page 29*
Neck stretches *page 30*
Knee bends *page 31*
Leg swings *page 31*

STANDING EXERCISES
Triceps kick-back *page 45*
Lateral leg raise *page 48*
Front leg raise *page 48*
Rear leg raise *page 49*

SEATED EXERCISES
Criss-cross arms *page 52*
Bent-over arm shaper *page 53*
Spine rotation *page 54*
Seated reverse abdominal curl *page 55*
Seated knee lift *page 56*
Simple seated thigh squeeze *page 57*
Seated leg extension *page 58*

COOL DOWN AND STRETCH
Standing waist stretch *page 86*
Sitting body twister *page 87*
Cobra stretch *page 89*
Knee hug *page 91*
Child's pose *page 91*

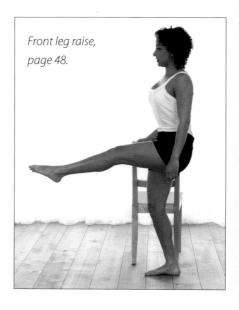

Front leg raise, page 48.

workout

INDEX

index

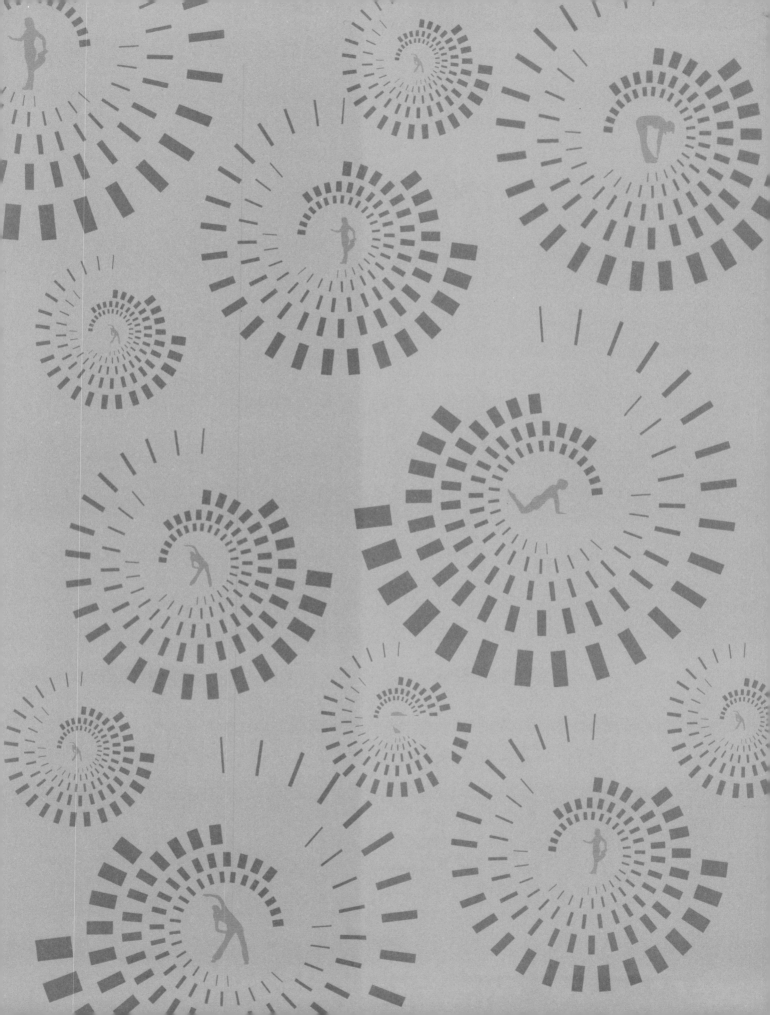